Fourth Edition

Study Guide to Accompany
Essentials of
Nursing Research
Methods, Appraisal, and Utilization

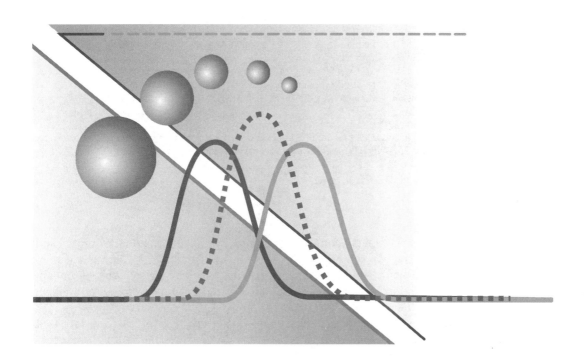

Acquisitions Editor: Margaret Zuccarini
Editorial Assistant: Emily Cotlier
Ancillary Editor: Doris S. Wray
Project Editor: Susan Deitch
Production Manager: Helen Ewan
Production Coordinator: Kathryn Rule
Design Coordinator: Kathy Kelley-Luedtke

Fourth Edition

9 8 7 6 5 4 3 2

ISBN: 0–397–55369–2

Care has been taken to confirm the accuracy of the information presented and to describe generally accepted practices. However, the authors, editors, and publisher are not responsible for errors or omissions or for any consequences from application of the information in this book and make no warranty, express or implied, with respect to the contents of the publication.

The authors, editors and publisher have exerted every effort to ensure that drug selection and dosage set forth in this text are in accordance with current recommendations and practice at the time of publication. However, in view of ongoing research, changes in government regulations, and the constant flow of information relating to drug therapy and drug reactions, the reader is urged to check the package insert for each drug for any change in indications and dosage and for added warnings and precautions. This is particularly important when the recommended agent is a new or infrequently employed drug.

Some drugs and medical devices presented in this publication have Food and Drug Administration (FDA) clearance for limited use in restricted research settings. It is the responsibility of the health care provider to ascertain the FDA status of each drug or device planned for use in their clinical practice.

Study Guide to Accompany
Essentials of
Nursing Research
Methods, Appraisal, and Utilization

Denise F. Polit, PhD

Humanalysis, Inc.
Saratoga Springs, New York
Formerly of the Boston College School of Nursing
Chestnut Hill, Massachusetts

Bernadette P. Hungler, RN, PhD

Boston College School of Nursing
Chestnut Hill, Massachusetts

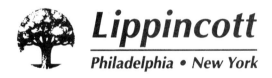

Lippincott
Philadelphia • New York

Preface

This study guide has been prepared to complement *Essentials of Nursing Research: Methods, Appraisal, and Utilization.* The guide provides opportunities to reinforce the acquisition of basic research skills through systematic learning exercises. The book is also intended to help bridge the gap between the passive reading of complex, abstract materials and the development of skills needed to evaluate research through concrete examples and study suggestions.

As in the case of the textbook, this study guide was developed on the premise that research examples are a critical component of the learning process. The inclusion of actual and fictitious research examples is designed to instruct (*i.e.*, facilitate the absorption of research concepts); motivate (*i.e.*, encourage students to envision the merit of acquiring research skills); and stimulate (*i.e.*, suggest topics that might be pursued further by nurse researchers and practicing nurses interested in the utilization of research findings).

This study guide consists of 14 chapters—one chapter corresponding to every chapter of the text. Each of the 14 chapters consists of five sections:

- *Matching Exercises*. Terms and concepts presented in the text are reinforced by having students perform a matching routine that often involves matching the concrete (*e.g.*, actual hypotheses) with the abstract (*e.g.*, types of hypotheses).
- *Completion Exercises*. Sentences are presented in which the student must fill in a missing word or phrase corresponding to important ideas presented in the text.
- *Study Questions*. Each chapter contains two to five short individual exercises relevant to the text materials, including the preparation of definition of terms.
- *Application Exercises*. These exercises are geared specifically to the consumers of nursing research and involve opportunities to critique various aspects of a study. Each chapter contains both fictitious research examples and suggestions for actual research reports, which students are asked to

evaluate according to a dimension emphasized in the corresponding chapter of the text. A new feature of this edition is the inclusion of two complete studies for students' critical appraisal.

- *Special Projects.* This section offers suggestions for fairly large projects in which, in many cases, an entire classroom could collaborate.

Contents

Overview of Nursing Research

PART I

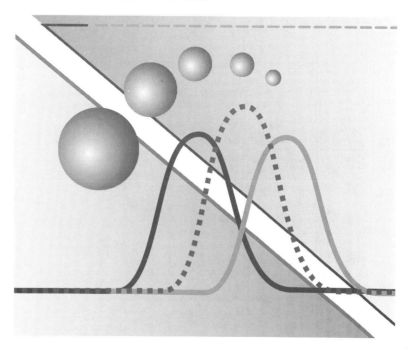

Chapter 1
Introduction to Nursing Research

◩ A. MATCHING EXERCISES

1. Match each of the activities in Set B with one of the time frames in Set A. Indicate the letter corresponding to the appropriate response next to each entry in Set B.

Set A

a. Pre-1950s
b. 1950s and 1960s
c. 1970s to present
d. None of the above

Set B   *Responses*

1. Nursing research focused on nurses themselves   _____
2. Increased research focus on clinical problems   _____
3. Establishment of the National Center for Nursing Research
   at the National Institutes of Health   _____
4. Creation of the professional journal *Research in Nursing
   and Health*   _____
5. First nursing research study was conducted   _____
6. Creation of the professional journal *Nursing Research*   _____
7. Increased interest in theoretical bases for conducting nursing
   research   _____
8. Federal funding becomes available to support nursing research   _____
9. Growing interest of nurse researchers in conducting in-depth,
   process-oriented studies   _____
10. Two professional nursing research journals cease publication
    due to low circulation   _____

2. Match each statement in Set B with one of the paradigms in Set A. Indicate the letter corresponding to the appropriate response next to each entry in Set B.

Set A

a. Positivist paradigm
b. Naturalist paradigm
c. Neither paradigm
d. Both paradigms

Set B   *Responses*

1. Assumes that reality exists and that it can be objectively studied and known   _____
2. Subjectivity in inquiries is considered inevitable and desirable   _____
3. Inquiries rely on external, empirical evidence that is collected through human senses   _____
4. Develops knowledge primarily through deductive processes   _____
5. Assumes reality is a construction and that many constructions are possible   _____
6. Relies primarily on the collection and analysis of quantitative information   _____
7. Relies primarily on the collection and analysis of narrative, qualitative information   _____
8. Provides a framework for inquiries undertaken by nurse researchers   _____
9. Inquiries give rise to emerging interpretations that are grounded in people's experiences   _____
10. Inquiries are not constrained by ethical issues   _____
11. Has its roots in 19th century philosophers such as Comte, Mill, Newton, and Locke   _____
12. Inquiries focus on discrete, specific concepts while attempting to control other aspects of a phenomenon   _____

◩ B. COMPLETION EXERCISES

Write the words or phrases that correctly complete the sentences below.

1. Research in nursing began with _____.
2. During the early years, most nursing studies focused on _____
   _____.
3. The rapid acceleration of nursing research began in the _____
   _____.
4. The future direction of nursing research is likely to involve a continuing focus on _____.
5. The most ingrained source of knowledge, and the one that is the most difficult to challenge, is _____.

6. The process of developing generalizations from specific observations is referred to as _____ reasoning.

7. The assumption that all phenomena have antecedent causes is called

_____.

8. The _____ paradigm is sometimes referred to as the phenomenologic or constructivist paradigm.

9. The traditional _____ approach to human knowledge uses systematic, controlled procedures to acquire information.

10. Evidence that is rooted in objective reality and gathered through the human senses is known as _____ evidence.

11. Because scientific inquiry is not concerned with isolated phenomena, a key goal of the scientific method is _____.

12. Researchers who reject the classical model of scientific inquiry criticize it for being overly _____.

13. Naturalistic inquiry always takes place in the _____

_____, in naturalistic settings.

14. The type of research that involves the systematic collection and analysis of controlled, numeric information is known as _____

_____.

15. The type of research that involves the systematic collection and analysis of subjective, narrative materials is known as _____

_____.

16. A specific aim of some qualitative research that asks "What is the name of this phenomenon?" is referred to as _____.

◨ C. STUDY QUESTIONS

1. Define the following terms. Use the textbook to compare your definition with the definition in Chapter 1 or in the Glossary.

a. Producer of nursing research: _____

_____

b. Consumer of nursing research: _____

_____

c. Journal club: _____

_____

d. National Institute of Nursing Research: _____

_____

  e. Assumption: _____

     _____

  f. Paradigm: _____

     _____

  g. Logical positivism: _____

     _____

  h. Generalizability: _____

     _____

  i. Applied research: _____

     _____

  j. Basic research: _____

     _____

2. Why is it important for nurses who will never conduct their own research to understand research methods?

3. What are some potential consequences to the profession of nursing if nurses stopped conducting their own research?

4. Students sometimes have concerns about courses on research methods. Complete the following sentences, expressing as honestly as possible your own feelings about research, and discuss your concerns with your class.

  a. I (am/am not) looking forward to this class on nursing research because:

     _____

     _____

  b. I think that I would like a course in nursing research methods better if:

     _____

     _____

  c. I think a class in nursing research (will/will not) improve my effectiveness as a nurse because:

     _____

     _____

5. Explain the ways in which knowledge from disciplined research differs from knowledge based on tradition, authority, trial and error, and logical reasoning.

6. How does the assumption of determinism conflict with or coincide with superstitious thinking? Take, as an example, the superstition associated with a four-leaf clover or a rabbit's foot.

7. Below are several research problems. For each, indicate whether you think it is *primarily* an applied or basic research question.

Research Question	*Type*
a. Does movement tempo affect perception of the passage of time?	_____
b. Does follow-up by nurses improve patients' compliance with their medication regimens?	_____
c. Does the ingestion of cranberry juice reduce urinary tract infections?	_____
d. Is sweat gland activity related to ACTH levels?	_____
e. Is pain perception associated with a person's locus of control (an aspect of personality)?	_____
f. Does the type of nursing curriculum affect attrition rates in schools of nursing?	_____
g. Does nicotine affect postural muscle tremor?	_____
h. Does the nurse/patient ratio affect nurses' job satisfaction?	_____

8. Below are descriptions of several research problems. Indicate whether you think the problem is best suited to a qualitative or quantitative approach, and indicate why you think this is so.
   a. What is the decision-making process of AIDS patients seeking treatment?

b. What effect does room temperature have on the colonization rate of bacteria in urinary catheters?

c. What is the nature of stress among nursing home residents?

d. Does therapeutic touch affect the vital signs of hospitalized patients?

e. What is the process by which nursing students acquire a professional nursing identity?

f. What are the effects of prenatal instruction on the labor and delivery outcomes of pregnant women?

g. What are the health care needs of the homeless, and what are the barriers they face in having those needs met?

9. What are some of the limitations of quantitative research? What are some of the limitations of qualitative research? Which approach seems best suited to address problems in which you might be interested? Why is that?

▧ D. APPLICATION EXERCISES

1. Below is a brief description of a fictitious study, followed by a critique. Do you agree with the critique? Can you add other comments relevant to issues discussed in Chapter 1 of the textbook? (Box 1-1 offers some guiding questions).

> ***Fictitious Study.*** *Lawrence and colleagues (1997) studied a sample of 100 nurses to determine whether the setting in which they practiced was related to their attitudes toward caring for patients with acquired immunodeficiency syndrome (AIDS). The settings chosen were acute hospital, hospice home care, clinics, and long-term care facilities. Each nurse completed a paper-and-pencil questionnaire comprising 20 questions. The questions asked them to rate (on a scale from 1 to 10) how important they considered physical care, help in dying, hope, protection of themselves, and other aspects of caring for AIDS patients. The researchers found that a higher percentage of nurses employed by acute care facilities believed that physical care and hope were important in caring for people with AIDS than did nurses employed in other settings. Nurses in all four types of settings identified protection of self as the most important aspect of care.*
>
> > ***Critique.*** *Although this study focused on a topic that is of great current interest, its relevance to nursing practice seems indirect. The researchers studied nurses' attitudes toward caring rather than focusing on actual nursing care. Studies examining problems encountered in the delivery of care, methods for helping patients with AIDS cope with the disease and death, or the timing of ministrations to reduce nausea or enhance nourishment would have been considerably more relevant to the practice of nursing. Studies focusing on people with AIDS are needed because of the ever-increasing number of people with the diagnosis. They represent a group with special needs and are a high-priority group for research inquiry. Redirecting the focus of the study to nursing care or to the needs of victims of this critical health problem would make it more useful. This brief abstract does not provide much information about the researcher's purpose and methodologic approach; however, it appears that Lawrence's study was quan-*

titative (for instance, she was able to compute percentages). The study described nurses' attitudes and explored the relation between attitudes and type of practice setting. The study generated some basic information about nurses' attitudes, but presumably the researcher intended to apply this knowledge in some fashion (e.g., to identify needs for training or education or to use the findings as a basis for discussions among nurses about caring for patients with AIDS).

2. Here is a brief summary of another fictitious study. Read the summary and then respond to the questions that follow.

Singleton (1996) studied the effect of the wording of communications on encouraging the elderly to come forward for a flu vaccination. All members of a senior citizens center in a midsized community (a total of 500 elderly men and women) were sent a letter advising them that a flu epidemic was anticipated that season and that the elderly were especially likely to benefit from an immunization. Half of the members were sent a letter stressing the benefits of getting a flu shot. The other half of the members were sent a letter stressing the potential dangers of not getting a flu shot. To avoid any biases, a lottery-type system was used to determine who got which letter. All of the elderly were advised that free immunizations would be available at a community health clinic over a 1-week period and that free transportation would also be made available to them. Singleton monitored the rates of coming forward for a flu shot among the two groups of elderly to assess whether one approach of encouragement was more persuasive than the other.

Consider the aspects of this study in relation to the issues discussed in this chapter. To assist you in your review, here are some guiding questions:
a. Discuss the relevance of this study to nursing.
b. Do the methods used in this study suggest that the underlying paradigm is positivism or naturalism? Would it be more appropriate to collect and analyze qualitative or quantitative information? Why do you think this is so?
c. How would you characterize the purpose of this study? Is its major aim description, exploration, explanation, prediction, or control? Is there more than one purpose?
d. Would you say this study is an example of basic or applied research?

3. Another brief summary of a fictitious study follows. Read the summary and then respond to questions a to d from Question D.2 in terms of this study.

Rimmer (1995) designed a study to explore and describe the meaning of the risk experience among middle-aged men and

*women whose parents had died of colon cancer and who
therefore were at elevated risk for colon cancer themselves.
A sample of 15 people whose parents had died within the previous 12 months were recruited for the study. In-depth interviews, lasting between 1 and 2 hours, were conducted in the
sample members' homes. The interviews were tape-recorded
and later transcribed. The interviews examined such issues
as perceptions of risk, factors contributing to the perceptions,
stress associated with risk perceptions, risk reduction efforts,
and coping strategies.*

4. Below are several suggested research articles. Skim one or more of these arti-
cles and respond to parts a to d of Question D.2 in terms of an actual research
study:
   - Admi, H. (1996). Growing up with a chronic health condition: A model of an
     ordinary lifestyle. *Qualitative Health Research, 6,* 163–183.
   - Craft, M. J., & Moss, J. (1996). Accuracy of infant emesis volume assess-
     ment. *Applied Nursing Research, 9,* 2–8.
   - Oehler, J. M., Thompson, R. J., Goldstein, R. F., Gustafson, K. E., & Brazy,
     J. E. (1996). Behavioral characteristics of very-low-birthweight infants of
     varying biologic risk at 6, 15, and 24 months of age. *Journal of Obstetric,
     Gynecologic, and Neonatal Nursing, 25,* 233–239.
   - Perry, J., & Olshansky, E. F. (1996). A family's coming to terms with
     Alzheimer's disease. *Western Journal of Nursing Research, 18,* 12–22.

◩ E. SPECIAL PROJECTS

1. Consider the following research statement:

   *The purpose of this study is to determine whether patients in
   intensive care units are or are not satisfied with their nursing
   care.*

   The basic purpose of this study as stated is descriptive. Alter the statement in
   such a way as to design a study whose essential purpose is exploration; explanation; prediction; and control.
2. Think of the last fact you learned with respect to clinical nursing practice. Try
   to discover the ultimate source of this information. Was it tradition ("this is the
   way it's always been done"); authorities ("Dr. So-and-so said so"); logical reasoning ("this has been inferred from previous observations"); or scientific
   method ("an empirical investigation discovered this to be the case")?

Chapter 2
Overview of the Research Process

◩ A. MATCHING EXERCISES

1. Match each of the terms in Set B with one of the responses in Set A. Indicate the letter corresponding to your response next to each item in Set B.

Set A

a. Term used in quantitative research
b. Term used in qualitative research
c. Term used in both qualitative or quantitative research

Set B   *Responses*

1. Subject   _____
2. Study participant   _____
3. Informant   _____
4. Variable   _____
5. Phenomena   _____
6. Construct   _____
7. Theory   _____
8. Data   _____

2. Match each of the terms in Set B with one (or more) of the terms in Set A. Indicate the letter corresponding to your response next to each item in Set B.

Set A

a. Categorical variable
b. Continuous variable
c. Constant

Set B   *Responses*

1. Employment status (working/not working)   _____
2. Dosage of a new drug   _____
3. Pi π (to calculate area of a circle)   _____
4. Number of aspirins ingested   _____

    5. Method of teaching patients (structured versus unstructured)   _____

    6. Blood type   _____

    7. pH level of urine   _____

    8. Pulse rate of a deceased person   _____

    9. Membership (versus nonmembership) in a nursing organization   _____

  10. Birth weight of an infant   _____

  11. Presence or absence of decubitus   _____

  12. Degree of empathy in nurses   _____

3. Match each of the terms in Set B with one of the terms in Set A. Indicate the letter corresponding to your response next to each item in Set B.

Set A

    a. Independent variable

    b. Dependent variable

    c. Either/both

Set B   *Response*

    1. The variable that is the presumed effect   _____

    2. The variable that is categorical   _____

    3. The variable that is the main outcome of interest in the study   _____

    4. The variable that is the presumed cause   _____

    5. The variable referred to as the criterion variable   _____

    6. The variable that is an attribute   _____

    7. The variable, "length of stay in hospital"   _____

    8. The variable that requires an operational definition   _____

◤ B. COMPLETION EXERCISES

Write the words or phrases that correctly complete the sentences below.

    1. The person who is the leader of a team of researchers is known as the _____ or _____.

    2. In a quantitative study, the people who are being studied in a research project are often referred to as the _____, but they may be referred to as the _____ in both qualitative and quantitative studies.

    3. The abstract qualities in which a researcher is interested are referred to by both qualitative and quantitative researchers as _____ _____.

4. A _____, a term used primarily in quantitative research, is a quality of a person, group, setting, or situation that takes on different values.

5. A _____ variable is one that takes on only a few discrete values.

6. The variable presumed to *cause* changes in some other variable is the _____ variable.

7. The variable that the researcher wants to understand, explain, or predict is known as the _____ variable.

8. If a researcher studied the effect of a scheduling assignment on nurses' morale, scheduling assignment would be referred to as the _____ variable.

9. The pieces of information obtained in the course of a study are collectively known as the _____.

10. When a quantitative researcher carefully specifies the steps that must be taken to measure the concepts of interest, the researcher develops _____.

11. When the data are in the form of narrative descriptions, the data are said to be _____.

12. Although quantitative researchers are often interested in studying relationships between variables, qualitative researchers examine _____.

13. "The higher the caloric intake, the greater the weight" expresses a presumed _____ relationship.

14. "Men are more likely to suffer depression after the death of their spouses than women" expresses a presumed _____ relationship.

15. When little is known about a topic or phenomenon, _____ research is likely to be more fruitful than _____ research.

16. There is typically a well-defined, pre-specified set of activities with fairly linear progression in a _____ study.

17. The overall plan for collecting and analyzing research data is called the _____.

18. The actual group of people selected from a larger group to participate in a study is known as the _____.

19. Typically, the most time-consuming phase of the study is the _____ phase.

20. The task of organizing and synthesizing the information collected in a study is known as _____.

21. A small-scale trial run of a research study is referred to as a(n) _____.

22. The findings from an investigation are communicated in a _____, which are most accessible to students in the form of _____.

23. The final phase of a research project is known as the _____ phase.

24. In a qualitative study, an important activity after identifying a research site is developing a strategy for _____ into selected settings within the site.

25. Quantitative researchers decide in advance how many study participants to include in a study, but qualitative researchers' sampling decisions are often guided by the principle of _____ of the data.

26. The six sections most often found in research journal articles are _____, _____, _____, _____, _____, and _____.

◧ C. STUDY QUESTIONS

1. Define the following terms. Use the textbook to compare your definition with the definition in Chapter 2 or in the Glossary.

   a. Informant: _____
   _____

   b. Construct: _____
   _____

   c. Operational definition: _____
   _____

   d. Variable: _____
   _____

   e. Attribute variable: _____
   _____

   f. Constant: _____
   _____

   g. Heterogeneity: _____
   _____

h. Relationship: _____

_____

i. Cause-and-effect relationship: _____

_____

j. Functional relationship: _____

_____

k. Population: _____

_____

l. Representativeness: _____

_____

m. Coding: _____

_____

n. Raw data: _____

_____

o. Research findings: _____

_____

p. "Blind" review: _____

_____

q. Abstract: _____

_____

r. Statistical tests: _____

_____

2. Suggest operational definitions for the following concepts.

a. Stress: _____

_____

b. Prematurity of infants: _____

_____

c. Nursing effectiveness: _____

_____

d. Prolonged labor: _____

_____

e. Nurses' job satisfaction: _____

_____

f. Respiratory function: _____

_____

3. In each of the following research problems, identify the independent variables and dependent variables.

a. Does assertiveness training improve the effectiveness of psychiatric nurses?

Independent: _____

Dependent: _____

b. Does the postural positioning of patients affect their respiratory function?

Independent: _____

Dependent: _____

c. Is the psychological well-being of patients affected by the amount of touch received from nursing staff?

Independent: _____

Dependent: _____

d. Is the incidence of decubitus reduced by more frequent turnings of patients?

Independent: _____

Dependent: _____

e. Is the educational preparation of nurses related to their subsequent turnover rate?

Independent: _____

Dependent: _____

f. Is tolerance for pain related to a patient's age and gender?

Independent: _____

Dependent: _____

g. Are the number of prenatal visits of pregnant women associated with labor and delivery outcomes?

Independent: _____

Dependent: _____

h. Are levels of stress among nurses higher in pediatric or adult intensive care units?

Independent: _____

Dependent: _____

i. Are student nurses' clinical grades related to their subsequent on-the-job performances?

Independent: _____

Dependent: _____

j. Is anxiety in surgical patients affected by structured preoperative teaching?
   Independent: _____
   Dependent: _____

k. Are nurses' promotions related to their level of participation in continuing education activities?
   Independent: _____
   Dependent: _____

l. Does hearing acuity of the elderly change as a function of the time of day?
   Independent: _____
   Dependent: _____

m. Is patient satisfaction with nursing care related to the congruity of nurses' and patients' cultural backgrounds?
   Independent: _____
   Dependent: _____

n. Is a woman's educational background related to breast self-examination practices?
   Independent: _____
   Dependent: _____

o. Does home birth affect the parents' satisfaction with the childbirth experience?
   Independent: _____
   Dependent: _____

4. For each of the variables in Question C.3, indicate which is a categorical variable and which is a continuous variable.

◪ D. APPLICATION EXERCISES

1. Below is a brief description of certain aspects of a fictitious study, followed by a critique. Do you agree with the critique? Can you add other comments relevant to issues discussed in Chapter 2 of the textbook? (Box 2-5 offers some guiding questions.)

> ***Fictitious Study.*** *Kaye (1996) studied factors affecting the duration of breastfeeding among low-income women living in an urban community. The factors under scrutiny were the*

mothers' educational attainment, their level of depression, and their race and ethnicity. The variables in the study were defined as follows:

- *Breastfeeding duration: The age of the child (in weeks) when he or she was totally weaned from the breast.*
- *Educational attainment: The highest grade in school that the mother completed.*
- *Level of depression: The mother's score on the Center for Epidemiological Studies Depression (CES-D) Scale.*
- *Race and ethnicity: Whether the mother was African American, white, or Hispanic.*

***Critique.** There are four concepts (variables) in Kaye's study. The dependent variable is breastfeeding duration, and the independent variables are educational attainment, level of depression, and race and ethnicity. Kaye is interested in knowing whether a mother's decision to prolong or curtail breastfeeding is related to how far she went in school, how depressed she is, and what her cultural background is.*

Although we do not have much information about the design of Kaye's study, we do know that she controlled at least two extraneous variables: socioeconomic status and area of residence. The study focused exclusively on low-income urban women; thus, income and urban residence were, in this study, not allowed to vary. Holding these variables constant enhanced Kaye's ability to interpret the results of her study.

Kaye's operational definitions appear to be reasonably good, but they could be expanded to indicate how the data would be collected. For example, for the dependent variable (breastfeeding duration), the definition might be the age of the child (in weeks) when he or she was totally weaned from the breast, as reported by the mother in an interview completed when the child was 2 years old.

2. Here is a brief description of certain aspects of another fictitious study. Read the description and then respond to the questions that follow.

Hebert (1996) observed that different patients react differently to sensory overload in the hospital. She conducted a study to see whether aspects of the patients' home environments (such as noise levels) affect their reactions to hospital noises. Below are the investigator's operational definitions of the research variables.

- *Type of home environment. Based on the patients' self-reports at intake, home environment was defined as the number of household members residing with the patient.*
- *Reaction to hospital noise. Based on responses to five questions answered at discharge, patients were classified as "dissatisfied with noise level" or "not dissatisfied with noise level."*

Review and comment on these specifications. To aid you in this task, here are some guiding questions:

a. What is the independent variable and what is the dependent variable in this study? Are these variables categorical or continuous?

b. Are the operational definitions sufficiently detailed? Do they tell you exactly how each variable is to be measured? Can you expand any of the definitions so that they are more precise?

c. Are the operational definitions good definitions—that is, is there a better way to measure the independent or dependent variables?

d. What type of relationship is implied by the research question—a functional or causal relationship?

e. This study was quantitative; is the question the researcher posed appropriate for a quantitative inquiry? Would a more qualitatively oriented approach have been more appropriate?

3. Below are several suggested research articles for quantitative studies. Read one of these articles and respond to parts a to e of Question D.2 in critiquing this actual research study. Also use the guidelines in Box 2-1 of the textbook to do a preliminary assessment of other aspects of the study.

- Beach, E. K., Maloney, B. H., Plocica, A. R., Sherry, S. E., Weaver, M., Luthringer, L., & Utz, S. (1992). The spouse: A factor in recovery after acute myocardial infarction. *Heart and Lung, 21,* 30–38.

- Dansky, K. H., Dellasega, C., Shellenbarger, T., & Russo, P. C. (1996). After hospitalization: Home health care for elderly persons. *Clinical Nursing Research, 5,* 185–198.

- DiIorio, C., Faherty, B., & Manteuffel, B. (1992). Self-efficacy and social support in self-management of epilepsy. *Western Journal of Nursing Research, 14,* 292–303.

- Fuller, B. F., Keefe, M. R., & Curtin, B. J. (1994). Acoustic analysis of cries from "normal" and "irritable" infants. *Western Journal of Nursing Research, 16,* 243–250.

4. A second brief description of a fictitious study follows. Read the description and then respond to the questions that follow.

Weiser (1997) undertook a study to understand the meaning of compliance with a medical regimen from the patient's perspective among low-income rural patients with a chronic health problem. Weiser noted that although compliance is a

*widely researched phenomenon, the patient's viewpoint is
often ignored. The researcher recruited a sample of 18 men
and women ranging in age from 27 to 68 from a health clinic
in rural Tennessee. The in-depth interviews, which lasted approximately 90 minutes on average, were conducted at the
clinic. The interviews focused on the nature of the chronic
health problem, the nature of the therapeutic regimen, and the
meaning of compliance from the informants' perspective.*

Review and comment on this study. To aid you in this task, here are some guiding questions.

  a. What is the central phenomenon under study in this research project?

  b. Is the question the researcher posed appropriate for a qualitative inquiry?
Would a more quantitatively oriented approach have been more appropriate?

  c. What types of patterns of association, if any, did the research explore?

  d. What is the setting for the study? Was this setting appropriate? How difficult do you think it was to gain entrée into this setting?

5. Below are several suggested research articles for qualitative studies. Read one
of these articles and respond to parts a to d of Question D.4 in critiquing this
actual research study. Also use the guidelines in Box 2-1 of the textbook to do
a preliminary assessment of other aspects of the study.

- Beck, C. T. (1996). Postpartum depressed mothers' experiences interacting
with their children. *Nursing Research, 45,* 98–109.

- Hamera, E. K., Pallikkathayil, L., Bauer, S., & Burton, M. R. (1994). Descriptions of wellness by individuals with schizophrenia. *Western Journal of
Nursing Research, 16,* 288–300.

- Milliken, P. J., & Northcott, H. C. (1996). Seeking validation: Hyperthy-
roidism and the chronic illness trajectory. *Qualitative Health Research, 6,*
202–223.

- Saveman, B., Hallberg, I. R., & Norberg, A. (1996). Narratives by district
nurses about elder abuse within families. *Clinical Nursing Research, 5,*
220–236.

▨ E. SPECIAL PROJECTS

1. Below is a list of variables. For each, think of a research problem for which the
variable would be the independent variable and a second for which it would be
the dependent variable. For example, take the variable "birth weight of infants." We might ask, "Does the age of the mother affect the birth weight of her
infant?" (dependent variable). Alternatively, we could define our research
question as, "Does the birth weight of infants (independent variable) affect
their sensorimotor development at 6 months of age?" HINT: For the dependent
variable problem, ask yourself, "What factors might affect, influence, or cause

this variable?" For the independent variable, ask yourself, "What factors might *this* variable influence, cause, or affect?"

a. Body temperature

Independent: _____

_____

Dependent: _____

_____

b. Amount of sleep

Independent: _____

_____

Dependent: _____

_____

c. Compliance with a medication regimen

Independent: _____

_____

Dependent: _____

_____

d. Level of hopefulness in patients

Independent: _____

_____

Dependent: _____

_____

e. Amount of saliva secretion

Independent: _____

_____

Dependent: _____

_____

2. Think of five pairs of variables that might have a relationship between them (*e.g.,* smoking status and lung cancer status). For each pair, indicate whether you presume the relationship to be functional or causal.

3. Suppose that a researcher wanted to do a qualitative study of a couple's decision to seek infertility treatment. What types of sites and settings might be appropriate for such a study? Describe some steps the researcher might have to take to gain entree into appropriate research settings.

Preliminary Steps in the Research Process

PART II

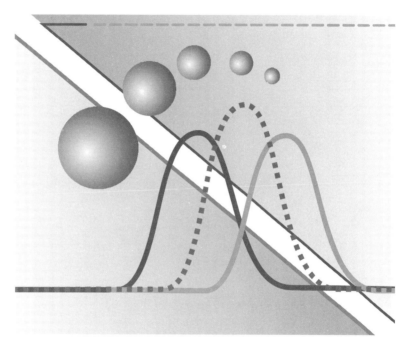

Chapter 3
Research Problems, Research Questions, and Hypotheses

▨ A. MATCHING EXERCISES

1. Match each of the research problems in Set B with one of the statements in Set A. Indicate the letter corresponding to the appropriate response next to each statement in Set B.

Set A

a. Statement of purpose—qualitative study
b. Statement of purpose—quantitative study
c. Not a statement of purpose for a research study

Set B   *Responses*

1. The purpose of this study is to test whether the removal of physical restraints affects behavioral changes in elderly patients.   _____
2. The purpose of this project is to facilitate the transition from hospital to home among women who have just given birth.   _____
3. The goal of this project is to explore the process by which an elderly person adjusts to placement in a nursing home.   _____
4. The investigation was designed to document the incidence and prevalence of smoking, alcohol use, and drug use among adolescents aged 12 to 14.   _____
5. The study's purpose was to describe the nature of touch used by parents in touching their preterm infants.   _____
6. The goal is to develop guidelines for spiritually related nursing interventions.   _____
7. The purpose of this project is to examine the relationship between race/ethnicity and the use of over-the-counter medications.   _____
8. The purpose is to develop an in-depth understanding of patients' feelings of powerlessness in hospital settings.   _____

2. Match each of the statements in Set B with one of the terms in Set A. Indicate the letter corresponding to the appropriate response next to each statement in Set B.

Set A

a. Research hypothesis—directional
b. Research hypothesis—nondirectional
c. Null hypothesis
d. Not a hypothesis as stated

Set B   *Responses*

1. First-born infants have higher concentrations of estrogens and progesterone in umbilical cord blood than do later-born infants.   _____
2. There is no relationship between participation in prenatal classes and the health outcomes of infants.   _____
3. Nursing students are increasingly interested in obtaining advanced degrees.   _____
4. Nurse practitioners have more job mobility than do other registered nurses.   _____
5. A person's age is related to his or her difficulty in accessing health care.   _____
6. Glaucoma can be effectively screened by means of tonometry.   _____
7. Increased noise levels result in increased anxiety among hospitalized patients.   _____
8. Media exposure of the health hazards of smoking is unrelated to the public's smoking habits.   _____
9. Patients' compliance with their medication regimens is correlated with their perceptions of the consequences of noncompliance.   _____
10. The primary reason that nurses participate in continuing education programs is for professional advancement.   _____
11. Baccalaureate, diploma, and associate degree nursing graduates differ with respect to technical and clinical skills acquired.   _____
12. A cancer patient's degree of hopefulness regarding the future is unrelated to his or her religiosity.   _____
13. The degree of attachment between children and their mothers is associated with the level of anxiety they experience during a hospitalization.   _____

14. The presence of homonymous hemianopia in stroke patients negatively affects their length of stay in the hospital.   _____

15. Adjustment to hemodialysis does not vary by the patient's gender.   _____

B. COMPLETION EXERCISES

Write the words or phrases that correctly complete the sentences below.

1. A _____ is a situation involving an enigmatic, puzzling, or disturbing condition that is of interest to a researcher.

2. A _____ is a statement of the specific query the researcher seeks to answer.

3. The accomplishments a researcher hopes to achieve by conducting a study are referred to as the _____ or _____.

4. The five most common sources of ideas for research problems are _____, _____ , _____, _____, and _____.

5. Research questions involving the essence, experience, process, or nature of some phenomenon would likely be addressed in a _____ study.

6. Unavailability of subjects would make a research project _____ _____.

7. Moral or philosophical questions are inherently _____.

8. Although it is desirable to have a statement of purpose placed early in a research report, the most typical location is at the end of the _____ _____.

9. Research hypotheses state a predicted _____ between variables.

10. A hypothesis involves a prediction regarding at least _____ variables.

11. A hypothesis that states a prediction regarding two or more independent and two or more dependent variables is called a _____ or _____ hypothesis.

12. The _____ hypothesis states that there is no expected relationship among the research variables.

◩ C. STUDY QUESTIONS

1. Define the following terms. Use the textbook to compare your definition with the definition in Chapter 3 or in the Glossary.

   a. Problem statement: _____

   _____

   b. Research aim: _____

   _____

   c. Statement of purpose: _____

   _____

   d. Hypothesis: _____

   _____

   e. Simple hypothesis: _____

   _____

   f. Complex hypothesis: _____

   _____

   g. Nondirectional hypothesis: _____

   _____

   h. Null hypothesis: _____

   _____

   i. Directional hypothesis: _____

   _____

2. Below is a list of general topics that could be investigated. Develop at least one research question for each, making sure that some are questions that could be addressed through qualitative research and others are ones that could be addressed through quantitative research. (HINT: For quantitative research questions, think of these concepts as potential independent or dependent variables; then ask, "What might cause or affect this variable?" and "What might be the consequences or effects of this variable?" This should lead to some ideas for research questions.)

   a. Patient comfort: _____

   _____

   b. Psychiatric patients' readmission rates: _____

   _____

   c. Anxiety in hospitalized children: _____

   _____

d. Student attrition from nursing school: _____

    _____

e. Attitudes toward artificial insemination: _____

    _____

f. Incidence of venereal disease: _____

    _____

g. Menstrual irregularities: _____

    _____

h. Requests for tubal ligation: _____

    _____

i. Elevated blood pressure: _____

    _____

j. Nurses' job satisfaction: _____

    _____

k. Patient cooperativeness in the recovery room: _____

    _____

l. Nutritional knowledge: _____

    _____

m. Mother–infant bonding: _____

    _____

3. Below is a list of research questions and statements of purpose. Transform those stated in the interrogative form (as research questions) to the declarative form (as statements of purpose), and vice versa.

Original Version   *Transformed Version*

a. Can a program of nursing counseling affect sexual readjustment among women after a hysterectomy?

b. The purpose of the research is to study the lived experience of parents whose young children have died of cancer.

c. What are the sequelae of an inadequately maintained sterile environment for tracheal suctioning?

Original Version	*Transformed Version*

d. What are the cues nurses use to determine pain in infants?

e. The purpose of the study is to investigate the effect of an AIDS education workshop on teenagers' understanding of AIDS and HIV.

f. The purpose of the research is to fully describe patients' responses to transfer from a coronary care unit.

g. What effect does the presence of the father in the delivery room have on the mother's satisfaction with the childbirth experience?

h. The purpose of the study is to explore why some women fail to perform breast self-examination regularly.

i. What is the long-term child development effect of maternal heroin addiction during pregnancy?

j. The purpose of the research is to study the effect of spermicides on the physiologic development of the fetus.

4. Below are five nondirectional hypotheses. Restate each one as a directional hypothesis.

Nondirectional	*Directional*

a. Nurses' attitudes toward mental retardation vary according to their clinical specialty area.

b. Nurses and patients differ in terms of the relative importance they attach to having the patients' physical versus emotional needs met.

c. Type of nursing care (primary versus team) is unrelated to patient satisfaction with the care they receive.

d. The incidence of decubitus ulcers is related to the frequency of turning patients.

e. Baccalaureate and associate degree nurses differ in use of touch as a therapeutic device with patients.

5. Below are five simple hypotheses. Change each one to a complex hypothesis by adding either a dependent variable or an independent variable.

Simple Hypothesis   *Complex Hypothesis*

a. First-time blood donors experience greater stress during the donation than donors who have given blood previously.

b. Nurses who initiate more conversation with patients are rated more effective in their nursing care by patients than those who initiate less conversation.

c. Surgical patients who give high ratings to the informativeness of nursing communications experience less preoperative stress than do patients who give low ratings.

d. Appendectomy patients whose peritoneums are drained with a Penrose drain experience more peritoneal infection than patients who are not drained.

e. Women who give birth by cesarean section are more likely to experience postpartum depression than women who give birth vaginally.

6. In Study Questions 4 and 5, 10 research hypotheses were provided. Identify the independent and dependent variables in each.

Independent Variable   *Dependent Variable*

4a. _____   _____

4b. _____   _____

4c. _____   _____

4d. _____   _____

4e. _____   _____

5a. _____   _____

5b. _____   _____

5c. _____   _____

5d. _____   _____

5e. _____   _____

D. APPLICATION EXERCISES

1. Below is a brief description of a research problem for a fictitious study, followed by a critique. Do you agree with the critique? Can you add other comments relevant to issues discussed in Chapter 3 of the textbook? (Box 3-1 offers some guiding questions).

Fictitious Study. Leighton (1996) was interested in studying nonverbal communication between nurses and patients. After some preliminary reading and discussions with colleagues, she decided to focus on touch as the medium of communication. She described her research question as follows: Does the amount of touching nurses give to patients affect the patients' recovery? Based on Leighton's readings regarding the effects of touch, she formulated the following hypotheses:

- *Without specific instruction regarding touching as a therapeutic form of communication, nurses do not engage in much touching behavior.*
- *The more nurses touch their patients, the higher the patients' morale.*
- *The greater the amount of physical contact between nurses and patients, the greater is the likelihood that the patients will comply with nurses' instructions, and the fewer the number of days of hospitalization.*

Critique. This example illustrates how the researcher narrowed and refined a broad topic of interest—nonverbal communication—and developed several research hypotheses in a series of steps. Those steps involved reviewing the literature, consulting with other nurses, identifying a specific area of interest for investigation, developing a research question, and finally, formulating the research hypotheses.

Using the criteria presented in this chapter, we can evaluate Leighton's research question and hypotheses. The research question appears to meet the criterion of significance: There are some tangible and important applications that can be made of the findings for the nursing profession. The question does not deal with a moral or ethical issue and meets the criterion for researchability. Without further information, we cannot judge the feasibility of the study, but presumably the study could be accomplished without undue constraints.

One difficulty, however, is that the leap between the research question and the hypotheses is a great one. The first hypothesis, though thematically related to the research question, does not address the issue of patient recovery at all. The second hypothesis is also tenuously connected to the problem statement; improved patient morale is undoubtedly a desirable outcome, but it is not really an acceptable way to operationalize speed of recovery. The final hypothesis (a complex hypothesis) is an appropriate translation of the formal problem statement into hypothesis form. Here, the researcher is defining patient recovery in terms of compliance with instructions and days spent in the hospital.

Aside from the gap between the research question and the hypotheses, there are additional problems with the hypotheses. The first hypothesis is untestable because it fails to state a predicted relationship between two variables. What criterion can we use to decide what "much touching" is? This hypothesis could be tested if rephrased in the following way: Nurses who receive instruction on the therapeutic value of touching will engage in more touching of patients than those who do not receive instruction.

In summary, there are many laudable features of Leighton's efforts. She has identified a significant, researchable topic and formulated some testable hypotheses; however, several modifications to the research question and hypotheses are in order.

2. Here is a brief description of certain aspects of another fictitious study. Read the description and then respond to the questions that follow.

Clain (1996) was interested in studying the notes made by various members of the health care team on patients' hospital charts. The investigator was concerned with several aspects of the chart in terms of its communication potential to various hospital personnel. She began her project with some general questions, such as: Are the nurses' entries on the patient chart used by other staff? Who is most likely to read nurses' entries on the patient chart? Are there particular types of medical conditions that encourage staff utilization of nurses' entries? Do particular types of entries encourage utilization?

Clain proceeded to reflect on her own experiences and observations relative to these issues and reviewed the literature to find whether other researchers had these problems. Based on her review and reflections, Clain developed the following hypotheses:

- *Nursing notes on patients' charts are referred to infrequently by hospital personnel.*
- *Physicians refer to nursing notes on the patients' charts less frequently than do other personnel.*

- *The use of nursing notes by physicians is related to the location of the notes on the chart.*
- *Nurses perceive that nursing notes are referred to less frequently than they are in fact referred to.*
- *Nursing notes are more likely to be referred to by hospital personnel if the patient has been hospitalized for more than 5 days than if the patient has been hospitalized for 5 or fewer days.*

Review and critique the hypotheses and the process of developing them. Suggest alternative wordings or supplementary hypotheses. To assist you, here are some guiding questions (see also the questions in Box 3-1 of the text):

a. Are all of the hypotheses testable as stated? What changes (if any) are needed to make all the hypotheses testable?

b. Are the hypotheses all consistent in format and style? That is, are they directional, nondirectional, or stated in the null form? Suggest changes, if appropriate, that would make them consistent.

c. Are the hypotheses reasonable (*i.e.,* logical and consistent with your own experience and observations)? Are the hypotheses significant (*i.e.,* do they have the potential to contribute to the nursing profession)?

d. Based on the general problem that the researcher identified, can you generate additional hypotheses that could be tested? Can you suggest modifications to the hypotheses to make them complex rather than simple (*i.e.,* introduce additional independent or dependent variables)?

3. Below are several suggested research articles. Read the introductory sections of one or more of these articles and identify the research questions and hypotheses. Respond to parts a to d of Question D.2 in terms of these actual research studies, and also answer relevant questions from Box 3-1 of the textbook.

- Barkman, S., & Lunse, C. P. (1994). The effect of early ambulation on patient comfort and delayed bleeding after cardiac angiogram. *Heart & Lung, 21,* 1–5.
- Pooler-Lunse, C., Barkman, A., & Bock, B. F. (1996). Effects of modified positioning and mobilization on back pain and delayed bleeding in patients who had received heparin and undergone angiography. *Heart & Lung, 25,* 117–123.
- Ronen, T., & Abraham, Y. (1996). Retention control training in the treatment of younger versus older enuretic children. *Nursing Research, 45,* 78–86,
- Torkelson, D. J., Anderson, R. A., & McDaniel, R. R. (1996). Interventions in response to chemically dependent nurses: Effect of context and interpretation. *Research in Nursing and Health, 19,* 153–162.

4. Examine a recent issue of a nursing research journal. Find a report for a quantitative study that fails to state a hypothesis. Given the research questions or purpose statement of the study, can you generate one or more hypotheses?

5. Another brief summary of a fictitious study follows. Read the summary and then respond to the questions that follow.

> *Werronen (1997), herself an asthmatic, noticed that when she experienced dyspnea she had a tendency to stop moving. A preliminary search of the literature on dyspnea suggested that there was relatively little research on how people with a chronic pulmonary disease react to and cope with the sensation of dyspnea. She conducted a qualitative study guided by a very general question—how is dyspnea experienced by people with a chronic pulmonary disorder? As she began to discuss this issue with study participants, Werronen noticed that people with the three most common types of disease—asthma, emphysema, and bronchitis—had developed somewhat different strategies for coping with dyspnea. On the basis of her in-depth interviews (and her observations of several study participants experiencing dyspnea), her final research questions evolved into the following:*
> - *What are the coping strategies used by patients with different chronic pulmonary diseases to deal with dyspnea?*
> - *What aspects of the dyspnea experience trigger different coping mechanisms?*
> - *What are the patterns of coping mechanism used by patients (i.e., what strategies are used in what order?)*

Review and critique the researcher's research questions. To assist you, here are some guiding questions:

a. Comment on the significance of the research problem for the nursing profession.

b. Does the research problem appear to be well suited to a qualitative approach?

c. Does the researcher's development of her research questions appear to have followed an appropriate process?

d. Are the research questions worded properly?

6. Below are several suggested research articles. Read the introductory sections of one or more of these articles and identify the research questions. Respond to parts a to d of Question D.5 in terms of these actual research studies and also answer relevant questions from Box 3-1 of the textbook.

- Ailinger, R. L., & Causey, M. E. (1995). Health concept of older Hispanic immigrants. *Western Journal of Nursing Research, 17,* 605–613.
- Conco, D. (1995). Christian patients' views of spiritual care. *Western Journal of Nursing Research, 17,* 266–276.
- Gibbins, S. A. M., & Chapman, J. S. (1996). Holding on: Parents' perceptions of premature infants' transfers. *Journal of Obstetric, Gynecologic, and Neonatal Nursing, 25,* 147–153.

- Hatton, D. C. (1994). Health perceptions among older urban American Indians. *Western Journal of Nursing Research, 16,* 392–403.

▧ E. SPECIAL PROJECTS

1. Read the article by Kuhlman and her colleagues (1991) entitled "Alzheimer's disease and family caregiving: Critical synthesis of the literature and research agenda," in *Nursing Research,* volume 40, issue 6 (or read some other research review article). Based on the authors' summary of prior research, develop a research question for a study that would extend our knowledge about Alzheimer's disease family caregiving. Assess your research question in terms of the criteria discussed in Chapter 3 of the textbook.

2. Below are five general topics that could be investigated. Develop two research questions for each—one that would lend itself to a qualitative inquiry and the other to a quantitative one. Assess the problem statement in terms of the criteria discussed in Chapter 3.

    a. Nurse–patient interaction: _____

    _____

    b. Bereavement: _____

    _____

    c. Nurses' diagnostic accuracy: _____

    _____

    d. Preoperative anxiety: _____

    _____

    e. Sleep disturbances: _____

    _____

3. Below are two sets of variables. Select a variable from each set to generate directional hypotheses. In other words, use one variable in Set A as the independent variable and one variable in Set B as the dependent variable (or vice versa), and make a prediction about the relationship between the two.* Generate five hypotheses in this fashion.

---

*As one example: Pregnant women who smoke will give birth to babies with lower Apgar scores than women who do not smoke.

Set A

Body temperature
Level of hopefulness
Attitudes toward death
Frequency of medications
Delivery by nurse midwife versus
    physician
Participation in prenatal education
    classes
Blood pressure
Amount of interaction between
    nurses and patients' families
Preoperative anxiety levels
Patients' amount of privacy during
    hospitalization
Smoking versus nonsmoking
Recidivism in a psychiatric hospital

Set B

Patient satisfaction with nursing care
Regular versus no exercise
Infant Apgar score
Patient gender
Effectiveness of nursing care
Patient capacity for self-care
Patients' compliance with nursing
    instructions
Amount of pain
Breastfeeding duration
Nurses' empathy
Patients' pulse rates
Length of stay in hospital

Chapter 4
Conceptual Contexts for Research Problems: Literature Reviews and Theoretical Frameworks

▧ A. MATCHING EXERCISES

1. Match each statement from Set B with one of the phrases in Set A. Indicate the letter corresponding to your response next to each of the statements in Set B.

Set A

a. Classic theory
b. Conceptual framework/model
c. Schematic model
d. Neither a, b, nor c
e. a, b, and c

Set B   *Responses*

1. Makes minimal use of language   _____
2. Uses concepts as building blocks   _____
3. Is essential in the conduct of good research   _____
4. Can be used as a basis for generating hypotheses   _____
5. Can be proved through empirical testing   _____
6. Indicates a system of propositions that assert relationships
   among variables   _____
7. Consists of interrelated concepts organized in a rational
   scheme but does not specify formal relationships among the
   concepts   _____
8. Exists in nature and is awaiting scientific discovery   _____

2. Match each conceptual framework/theory from Set B with one of the theorists in Set A. Indicate the letter corresponding to your response next to each of the statements in Set B.

Set A

a. Orem
b. Pender
c. Azjen-Fishbein
d. Becker
e. Lazarus-Folkman
f. Mishel

Set B   *Response*

1. Theory of Reasoned Action   _____
2. Health Belief Model   _____
3. Uncertainty in Illness Theory   _____
4. Model of Self-Care   _____
5. Theory of Stress and Coping   _____
6. Health Promotion Model   _____

◪ B. COMPLETION EXERCISES

Write the words or phrases that correctly complete the sentences below.

1. For nurses, the most widely used electronic database is _____.

2. Most electronic searches are likely to begin with a _____ search.

3. An electronic search that looks for a topic or keyword as it appears in the text fields of a record is referred to as a _____ search.

4. The two major types of print resources for a bibliographic search are _____ and _____.

5. In the context of the research literature, a _____ source is a description of a study written by the researchers who conducted it.

6. The two types of information that have the least utility in a research review are _____ and _____.

7. The most important type of information to be included in a written research review is _____.

8. Quantity of references is less important in a good literature review than the _____ of the references.

9. The written literature review should paraphrase materials and use a minimum of _____.

10. The literature review should make clear not only what is known about a problem but also any _____ in the research.

11. The review should conclude with a _____.

12. The literature review should be written in a language of _____ _____, in keeping with the limits of existing methods.

13. In a research report, a brief literature review is usually included in the _____, but in a qualitative study, the review may be presented in the _____ section.

14. A _____ is the conceptual underpinnings of a study.

15. Theories are not found by scientists, they are _____.

16. Most of the conceptualizations of nursing practice would be called _____ _____.

17. Schematic models attempt to represent reality with a minimal use of _____ _____.

18. The four central concepts of conceptual models in nursing are _____, _____, _____, and _____.

19. The acronym HPM stands for the _____.

20. Theoretical frameworks from nonnursing disciplines are sometimes referred to as _____.

▧ C. STUDY QUESTIONS

1. Define the following terms. Use the textbook to compare your definition with the definition in Chapter 4 or in the Glossary.

   a. Literature review: _____
   _____

   b. Mapping: _____
   _____

   c. Secondary source: _____
   _____

   d. Key word: _____
   _____

   e. Descriptive theory: _____
   _____

   f. Conceptual definition: _____
   _____

   g. Conceptual model: _____

              _____

   h. Schematic model: _____

              _____

   i. Middle-range theory: _____

              _____

2. Below are fictitious excerpts from literature reviews. Each excerpt has a stylistic problem for a research review. Change each sentence to make it acceptable stylistically.

Original	*Revised*

a. Most elderly people do not eat a balanced diet.

b. Patient characteristics have a significant impact on nursing workload.

c. A child's conception of appropriate sick role behavior changes as the child grows older.

d. Home birth poses many potential dangers.

e. Multiple sclerosis results in considerable anxiety to the family of the patient.

f. Studies have proved that most nurses prefer not to work the night shift.

g. Life changes are the major cause of stress in adults.

h. Stroke rehabilitation programs are most effective when they involve the patients' families.

i. It has been proved that psychiatric outpatients have higher than normal rates of accidental deaths and suicides.

j. Nursing faculty are increasingly involved in conducting their own research.

k. Sickle cell counseling has emerged as an important service in community health centers.

l. The traditional pelvic examination is sufficiently unpleasant to many women that they avoid having the examination.

Original	*Revised*

m. It is known that most tonsillectomies performed two decades ago were unnecessary.

n. Few smokers seriously try to break the smoking habit.

o. Severe cutaneous burns often result in hemorrhagic gastric erosions.

3. Below are several research questions. Indicate one or more terms or key words that you would use to begin a subject search on this topic.

Problem Statement	*Key Words*

a. How effective are nurse practitioners versus pediatricians with respect to telephone management of acute pediatric illness? _____

b. Does contingency contracting improve patient compliance with a treatment regimen? _____

c. What is the decision-making process for a woman considering having an abortion? _____

d. Is the amount of money a person spends on food related to the adequacy of nutrient intake? _____

e. Is rehabilitation after spinal cord injury affected by the age and social class of the patient? _____

f. Does the leadership style of head nurses affect the job tension and job performance of the nursing staff? _____

g. What is the course of appetite loss among cancer patients undergoing chemotherapy? _____

h. What is the effect of alcohol skin preparation before insulin injection on the incidence of local and systemic infection? _____

4. Read Susan Kelley's (1990) study entitled "Parental stress response to sexual abuse and ritualistic abuse of children in day care centers," which appeared in *Nursing Research, 39,* pages 25–29. Write a summary of the problem, methods, findings, and conclusions of the study. Your summary should be capable of serving as notes for a review of the literature on child abuse by child care providers.

5. Read some recent issues of *Nursing Research* or another nursing research journal. Identify at least two different theories cited by nurse researchers in these research reports.

6. Choose one of the conceptual frameworks or theories that were described in this chapter. Develop a research hypothesis based on this framework.

▧ D. APPLICATION EXERCISES

Below is a brief description of the literature review from a fictitious study by Nicolet (1996), followed by a critique. Do you agree with the critique? Can you add other comments relevant to issues relating to a literature review, as discussed in Chapter 4 of the textbook? (Box 4-1 offers some guiding questions.)

> ***Fictitious Literature Review.*** *There is now abundant evidence in the medical and epidemiologic literature that adolescents are at especially high risk of pregnancy complications, giving birth to low-birth-weight infants, and neonatal deaths (Hillard, 1982; Travis, 1986; Brown, 1983).* Relatively few studies, however, have examined the health status of children born to adolescent mothers after the first few weeks of life. The limited data that are available suggest that children of young mothers continue to be at a disadvantage throughout their infancy and later childhood. For example, Bradley and Lewis (1981) reported that the health of infants born to African American teenaged mothers was worse than that for infants of older African American mothers; particular problems were noted with respect to hypoglycemia, respiratory distress syndrome, pneumonia, and seizures. Hughes (1984), in her intensive study of young-parent families, reported an extremely high incidence of health problems among the infants: one fifth*

---

*All references in this example are fictitious, and the findings summarized here are not necessarily accurate.

had been hospitalized by the time they were 18 months old. According to Tilmon (1979), "These young women are simply not capable of attending to the needs of their children until these problems are so severe they require hospitalization" (p. 315).

Other investigators have proved that accidents and injuries are more prevalent among infants born to teenaged mothers. For example, Wright (1982) reported that the risk of infant accidental death was highest among mothers between 15 and 19 years of age. Similarly, Kestecher and Dickinson (1983) found that the most important difference in the health status between 3-year-old children with teenaged mothers was the high incidence of injuries and burns to those children with younger mothers.

Few empirical studies have attempted to unravel the factors that might lead to impaired health among the children born to younger mothers. The purpose of this study was to further our understanding of the factors that might lead to greater health problems and less appropriate use of health care among children born to adolescent mothers.

Critique. *For the most part, Nicolet appears to have done a fairly good job of organizing and briefly summarizing information about the effect of maternal age on an infant's health status. The research cited appears to be relevant to the research problem, and Nicolet seems to have relied on primary sources. Without doing a literature review ourselves, it would be difficult to know whether this review is accurate and thorough. We do know, however, that most of the references were fairly old. None of the research cited was conducted in the 3 years preceding publication of Nicolet's report. It is therefore likely that this review excluded other, more recent research on this topic—research that might have made a difference in Nicolet's conclusions and formulation of the problem.*

Nicolet's review can also be criticized for being fairly superficial. True, in journal articles, it is common for researchers to be succinct and to cite only the most important relevant studies. It would have been helpful, however, for Nicolet to make a statement about the believability of the previous research findings based on an assessment of the quality and integrity of the studies.

Two other points about the literature review merit comment. The first is that Nicolet inappropriately claimed that prior studies "proved" that accidents and injuries are more

prevalent among infants of young mothers. The word proved
should be changed to found *or some other tentative phrasing.*
Second, there is an irrelevant and subjective quotation buried
in a review that otherwise seems to be objective and neutral.
The quote by Tilmon does not belong in this review. At least
Nicolet should have introduced the quote this way: "Findings
such . . . as these have led some authorities to speculate about
whether young mothers are developmentally prepared to han-
dle the parenting role. For example, Tilmon (1979), who
chaired a panel on high-risk infants, made the comment . . ."

2. Below is a brief description of the conceptual framework used in the fictitious
   study by Nicolet (see exercise D.1 for her literature review). Do you agree with
   the critique that follows the description of the framework? Can you add other
   comments on the conceptual framework based on material covered in Chapter
   4 of the textbook? (Box 4-2 offers some guiding questions.)

   Fictitious conceptual framework. *The theoretical framework*
   for this study was the Health Belief Model (HBM). This model
   postulates that health-seeking behavior is influenced by the
   perceived threat posed by a health problem and the perceived
   value of actions designed to reduce the threat (Becker, 1978).
   Within the HBM, perceived susceptibility refers to a person's
   perception that a health problem is personally relevant. It is
   hypothesized that young mothers are developmentally unable
   to perceive their own (or their infant's) susceptibility to
   health risk accurately. Furthermore, adolescent mothers are
   hypothesized to be less likely, because of their developmental
   immaturity, to perceive accurately the severity of their in-
   fants' health problems and less likely to assess accurately the
   benefit of appropriate interventions than older mothers. Fi-
   nally, teenaged mothers are expected to evaluate less accu-
   rately the costs (which, in the HBM, include the complexity,
   duration, accessibility, and financial costs) of securing treat-
   ment. In summary, the HBM provides an excellent vehicle for
   testing the mechanisms through which children of young
   mothers are at higher-than-average risk of severe health prob-
   lems and are less likely to receive appropriate health care.

   Critique. *The theoretical basis for Nicolet's study was a*
   nonnursing model that has frequently been applied to prob-
   lems relating to health care use. This model appears to have
   provided an appropriate conceptual basis for the study. Al-
   though Nicolet might have provided somewhat more informa-
   tion regarding features of the HBM, she did explain the HBM
   sufficiently to clarify the basis for her hypotheses. Her hy-

potheses are clearly linked to the model and appear to be logically related to the problem at hand.

Previous research had yielded descriptive information suggesting that children born to teenaged mothers are at higher risk than other children for health problems and inadequate health care. By basing this research on the HBM, Nicolet was attempting to explain why this might be so. She hypothesized that the differences between the children of older and younger mothers reflect the younger mothers' appraisals of their children's needs and of the value of obtaining treatment. By operationalizing the key concepts in the HBM (e.g., perceived susceptibility, perceived severity of the illness, perceived cost of securing treatment), Nicolet's hypotheses can be put to an empirical test. If Nicolet found differences between older and young mothers in their appraisals of their children's health care needs, progress would have been made toward explaining differences in the children's health outcomes. If, however, Nicolet found no differences in mothers' appraisals, another researcher interested in the same problem would have to evaluate whether a different conceptual framework might be more productive in helping to explain differences in children's health and health care, or whether Nicolet failed—through her research design decisions—to test the HBM adequately.

3. Below is an excerpt from a fictitious literature review by Forester (1997) dealing with pelvic inflammatory disease. Read the literature review and then respond to the questions that follow.

There are no universally accepted criteria for defining pelvic inflammatory disease (PID) or for categorizing its severity. Furthermore, PID does not exhibit uniformity in its clinical features. Etiologically, cases of acute PID can be divided on the basis of those caused by Neisseria gonorrhoeae, *those caused by nongonococcal bacteria, and those caused by a combination of both. Eschenbach and his colleagues (1980) have reported that approximately half of the women with PID whom they examined had gonococcal infections. Eschenbach (1984) has noted that "this difference in etiological agents may explain the clinical differences between the gonococcal and nongonococcal PID. The latter may appear less acute and may not demonstrate many of the well-defined clinical features associated with gonorrhea" (p. 148). Both gonococcal and nongonococcal PID may result in subsequent obstruction of the fallopian tubes, which is among the most common causes of infertility in women. Because fertilized eggs remain in the fallopian tubes for approximately 3 days, they must provide nourishment for the developing zygote. Thus, even a tube that is not completely blocked, but that is severely damaged, can contribute to infertility.*

Westrom (1980), in a study of women treated for PID, proved that PID has an impact on subsequent fertility. A sample of 415 women with laparoscopically confirmed PID were reviewed after 9.5 years and compared with 100 control subjects who had never been treated for PID. Among the 415 women who had had PID, 88 (21.2%) were involuntarily childless; of these 88, the failure to conceive was due to tubal obstruction in 72 cases (82%). A total of 263 of the 415 subjects (63.4%) had become pregnant. In the control group, only three women (3%) were involuntarily childless.

Westrom's study also showed a relationship between infertility and the number of PID infections. Tubal occlusion was diagnosed after one infection in 32 women (12.8%); after two infections in 22 cases (35.5%); and after three or more infections in 18 cases (75.5%). Of the 415 women with acute PID in Westrom's sample, 94 (22.7%) experienced more than one infection. Evidence from other studies confirms that a large percentage of women with PID have a history of previous PID and that recurrent PID usually has a nongonococcal cause (Jacobson & Westrom, 1984; Ringrose, 1980; Eschenbach, 1981).

The number of women affected by PID annually in the United States is unknown and difficult to estimate. According to Rose (1986), Eschenbach and colleagues used data from the National Disease and Therapeutic Index Study and the Hospital Record Study to estimate that over 500,000 cases of PID occurred annually in the United States in the early 1980s. The information from the Hospital Record Study indicated that a mean of more than 160,000 patients with PID were hospitalized annually from 1980 through 1983.

Critique this literature review in regard to the points made in Chapter 4 of the textbook. To assist you in this task, you can answer the guiding questions that follow the review, as well as the applicable questions in Box 4-1 of the textbook.

a. Is the review well organized? Does the author skip from theme to theme in a disjointed way, or is there a logic to the order of presentation of materials?

b. Is the content of the review appropriate? Does the author use secondary sources when a primary source was available? Are all of the references relevant, or does the inclusion of some material appear contrived? Do you have a sense that the author was thorough in uncovering all of the relevant materials? Do the references seem outdated? Is there an overdependence on opinion articles or anecdotes? Are prior studies merely summarized, or are their shortcomings discussed? Does the author indicate what is not known as well as what is?

c. Does the style seem appropriate for a research review? Does the review seem biased or laden with subjective opinions? Is there too little paraphrasing and too much quoting? Does the author use appropriately tentative language in describing the results of earlier studies?

4. Read the literature review section in one of the articles listed below. Critique the review, applying parts a to c of Question D.3 as well as the questions in Box 4-1 of the textbook.

- Green, L. A., & Froman, R. D. (1996). Blood pressure measurement during pregnancy: Auscultatory versus oscillatory methods. *Journal of Obstetric, Gynecologic, and Neonatal Nursing, 25,* 155–159.
- Kennard, M. J., *et al.* (1996). Participation of nurses in decision making for seriously ill adults. *Clinical Nursing Research, 5,* 199–219.
- Marion, L. N., & Cox, C. L. (1996). Condom use and fertility among divorced and separated women. *Nursing Research, 45,* 110–115.
- Rutman, D. (1996). Caregiving as women's work: Women's experiences of powerfulness and powerlessness as caregivers. *Qualitative Health Research, 6,* 90–111.

5. Below is a description of the conceptual framework for another fictitious study. Read the summary and then respond to the questions that follow.

Sterling (1996) developed a study derived from Rotter's social learning theory. Social learning theory postulates that human behaviors are contingent on the individual's expectancy that a particular behavior will be reinforced (rewarded). A key concept is locus of control, which is conceptualized as the degree to which a person perceives that rewards are a function of his or her own actions as opposed to external forces. Internal controllers are those who perceive themselves and their behaviors as the major determinants of the reinforcement, and external controllers are those who tend to see little, if any, relationship between their own actions and subsequent reinforcement.

Sterling hypothesized that people with an internal locus-of-control orientation would be more likely to engage in preventive health care activities than those with an external ori-

entation. As a rationale for this hypothesis, she reasoned that internally oriented people see themselves as capable of controlling health outcomes, whereas externally oriented people see forces outside their control as the major determinants of health outcomes. Therefore, the externally oriented are less likely to engage in preventive health care behaviors. To test her hypothesis, Sterling operationalized "willingness to engage in preventive health care activities" as enrollment in a health maintenance organization among a group of employees who were offered a choice between a traditional medical benefits package and HMO membership. Five hundred employees hired by a large industrial firm were administered a test that measured locus of control as part of the application process. Each new employee was offered a choice between the two medical programs. The 187 employees who chose HMO membership were found to have significantly higher (i.e., more internal) scores on the locus-of-control measure than the 313 employees who elected the traditional medical plan, thereby supporting Sterling's hypothesis.

Review and critique the above study with respect to its theoretical basis. To assist you in this task, you can answer the guiding questions below as well as the questions in Box 4-2 of the text.

a. In what way, if any, did the use of a theory enhance the value of this study? Compare the meaningfulness of the study as described with what it would have been had the same hypothesis been tested in the absence of a theory.

b. In what way, if any, did the outcome of the study affect the value of the theory? If the outcome had been different (*e.g.*, no differences, or differences opposite to those predicted), what effect would that have had on the theory?

c. In the textbook, alternative ways of linking theory and research were described. In this example, how was the theory linked to the research?

6. Read the introductory sections of one of the actual research studies cited below. Apply parts a to c of Question D.5 to one of these studies as well as the questions in Box 4–2 of the textbook.

- Ajijevych, K., & Bernard, L. (1994). Health-promoting behaviors of African American women. *Nursing Research, 43*, 86–89.

- Brown, S. J. (1992). Tailoring nursing care to the individual client: Empirical challenge of a theoretical concept. *Research in Nursing and Health, 15*, 39–46.

- Coward, D. D. (1996). Self-transcendence and correlates in a healthy population. *Nursing Research, 45*, 116–121.

- Howell, S. L. (1994). A theoretical model for caring for women with chronic nonmalignant pain. *Qualitative Health Research, 4*, 94–122.

▧ E. SPECIAL PROJECTS

1. Read the literature review section from a research article appearing in an issue of *Nursing Research* in the 1980s (some possibilities are suggested below). Search the literature for more recent research on the topic of the article and update the review section. Do not forget to incorporate in your review the findings from the article itself! Here are some possible articles:
   - Austin, J. K., McBride, A. B., & Davis, H. W. (1984). Parental attitude and adjustment to childhood epilepsy. *Nursing Research, 33,* 92–96.
   - Hutchinson, S. A. (1987). Toward self-integration: The recovery process of chemically dependent nurses. *Nursing Research, 36,* 339–343.
   - Keane, A., Ducette, J., & Adler, D. (1985). Stress in ICU and non-ICU nurses. *Nursing Research, 34,* 231–236.
   - Kemp, V. H., & Hatmaker, D. D. (1989). Stress and social support in high-risk pregnancy. *Research in Nursing and Health, 12,* 331–336.
2. Select one of the problem statements from Question C.3. Conduct a literature search and identify 5 to 10 relevant references. Compare your references with those of your classmates in terms of relevance, recency, and type of information provided.
3. One proposition of reinforcement theory is that *if* a behavior is rewarded (reinforced), *then* the behavior will be repeated (learned). Based on this theory and on your observation of behaviors in health settings or schools of nursing, suggest three nursing research problem statements.
4. Develop a researchable problem statement based on Orem's Model of Self-Care.

Chapter 5
The Ethical Context of Nursing Research

◩ A. MATCHING EXERCISES

1. Match each of the descriptions in Set B with one of the procedures used to safeguard human subjects from Set A. Indicate the letter corresponding to the appropriate response next to each entry in Set B.

Set A

a. Freedom from harm or exploitation
b. Informed consent
c. Anonymity
d. Confidentiality

Set B   *Responses*

1. A questionnaire distributed by mail bears an identification number in one corner. Respondents are assured their responses will not be individually divulged.   _____

2. Hospitalized children included in a study, and their parents, are told the aims and procedures of the research. Parents are asked to sign an authorization.   _____

3. Respondents in a questionnaire study, in which the same respondents will be questioned twice, are asked to place their own four-digit identification number on the question-naire and to memorize the number. Respondents are assured that their answers will remain private.   _____

4. Study participants in an in-depth study of family members' coping with a natural disaster renegotiate the terms of their participation at successive interviews.   _____

5. Women who recently had mastectomies are studied in terms of psychological sequelae. In the interview, sensitive questions are carefully worded. After the interview, debriefing with the respondent determines the need for psychological support.   _____

6. Women interviewed in the above study (question 5) are told that the information they provide will not be individually divulged. _____

Set B   ***Responses***

7. Subjects who volunteered for an experimental treatment for AIDS are warned of potential side effects and are asked to sign a waiver.   _____

8. After determining that a new intervention resulted in discomfort to subjects, the researcher discontinued the study.   _____

9. Unmarked questionnaires are distributed to a class of nursing students. The instructions indicate that the responses will not be individually divulged.   _____

10. The researcher assures subjects that they will be interviewed as part of the study at a single point in time and adheres to this promise.   _____

11. A questionnaire distributed to a sample of nursing students includes a statement indicating that completion and submission of the questionnaire will be construed as voluntary participation in a study, as fully described in an accompanying letter.   _____

12. The names, ages, and occupations of study participants whose interviews are excerpted in the research report are not divulged.   _____

◩ B. COMPLETION EXERCISES

Write the words or phrases that correctly complete the sentences below.

1. Ethical _____ arise when the rights of subjects and the demands of science are put into direct conflict.

2. One of the first internationally recognized efforts to establish ethical standards was the _____.

3. The National Commission for the Protection of Human Subjects of Biomedical and Behavioral Research issued a well-known set of guidelines known as the

   _____.

4. The most straightforward ethical precept is the protection of subjects from

   _____.

5. Risks that are no greater than those ordinarily encountered in daily life are referred to as _____.

6. The right to _____ means that prospective subjects have the right to voluntarily decide whether to participate in a study, without risk of penalty.

7. The researcher adheres to the principle of _____ by fully describing to subjects the nature of the study and the likely risks and benefits of participation.

8. When the researcher cannot link research information to the person who provided it, the condition known as _____ has prevailed.

9. Special procedures are often required to safeguard the rights of _____ _____ subjects.

10. Committees established in institutions to review proposed research procedures with respect to their adherence to ethical guidelines are often called IRBs, or _____.

▨ C. STUDY QUESTIONS

1. Define the following terms. Use the textbook to compare your definition with the definition in Chapter 5 or in the Glossary.

   a. Code of ethics: _____
   _____

   b. Beneficence: _____
   _____

   c. Stipends: _____
   _____

   d. Debriefing: _____
   _____

   e. Risk/benefit ratio: _____
   _____

   f. Process consent: _____
   _____

   g. Coercion: _____
   _____

   h. Covert data collection: _____
   _____

   i. Deception: _____
   _____

   j. Confidentiality: _____
   _____

   k. Informed consent: _____
   _____

   l. Vulnerable subjects: _____
   _____

m. Implied consent: _____
_____

2. Below are descriptions of several research studies. Suggest some ethical dilemmas that might emerge for each.

a. An in-depth study of coping behaviors among rape victims:
_____
_____

b. An unobtrusive observational study of fathers' behaviors in the delivery room:
_____
_____

c. An interview study of the antecedents of heroin addiction:
_____
_____

d. An investigation of the contraceptive decisions of adolescents (minors) using a family planning clinic:
_____
_____

e. An investigation of the verbal interactions among schizophrenic patients:
_____
_____

f. A study of the effects of a new drug on human subjects:
_____
_____

3. The following two studies involved the use of vulnerable subjects. Evaluate the ethical aspects of one or both of these studies, paying special attention to the manner in which the subjects' heightened vulnerability was handled.

- Archbold, P. G., Stewart, B. J., Greenlick, M. R., & Harvath, T. (1990). Mutuality and preparedness as predictors of caregiver role strain. *Research in Nursing and Health, 13,* 375–383.
- Nyamathi, A. M. (1991). Relationship of resources to emotional distress, somatic complaints, and high-risk behaviors in drug recovery and homeless minority women. *Research in Nursing and Health, 14,* 269–277.

4. In Chapter 5 of the textbook, two unethical studies were described (the study of syphilis among black men and the study in which live cancer cells were injected in elderly patients). Identify which ethical principles were transgressed in these studies.

5. A stipend of $5.00 was paid to the subjects completing a questionnaire on breastfeeding in the following study: Hill, P. D. (1991). Predictors of breastfeeding duration among WIC and non-WIC mothers. *Public Health Nursing, 8,* 46–52.

    Read the introductory sections of the report and comment on the appropriateness of the stipend.

6. Comment on the risk/benefit ratio and other ethical aspects of the following study, in which a mild form of deception was used: Forrester, D. A. (1990). AIDS-related risk factors, medical diagnosis, do-not-resuscitate orders and aggressiveness of nursing care. *Nursing Research, 39,* 350–354.

▧ D. APPLICATION EXERCISES

1. Below is a brief description of the ethical aspects of a fictitious study, followed by a critique. Do you agree with the critique? Can you add other comments relevant to the ethical dimensions of the study (Box 5-2 of the textbook offers some guiding questions).

    Fictitious Study. *Godine (1997) conducted an in-depth study of nursing home patients to determine if their perceptions about personal control over decision making differed from the perceptions of the nursing staff. The investigator studied 25 nurse–patient dyads to determine whether there were differing perceptions and experiences regarding control over activities of daily living, such as arising, eating, and dressing. All of the nurses in the study were employed by the nursing home in which the patients resided. Because the nursing home had no IRB, Godine sought permission to conduct the study from the nursing home administrator. She also obtained the consent of the legal guardian or responsible family member of each patient. All study participants were fully informed about the nature of the study. The researcher assured the nurses and the legal guardians and family members of the patients of* *the confidentiality of the information and obtained their consent in writing. Data were gathered primarily through in-depth interviews with the patients and the nurses, at separate times. The researcher also observed interactions between the patients and nurses. The findings from the study showed that patients perceived that they had more control over all aspects of the activities of daily living (except eating) than the nurses perceived that they had. Excerpts from the interviews were used verbatim in the research report, but Godine did not divulge the location of the nursing home, and she used fictitious names for all participants.*

    Critique. *Godine did a reasonably good job of adhering to basic ethical principles in the conduct of her research. She obtained written permission to conduct the study from the nursing home administrator, and she obtained informed consent from the nurse participants and the legal guardians or family members of the patients. The study participants were not put at risk in any way, and the patients who participated may actually have enjoyed the opportunity to have a conversation with the researcher. Godine also took appropriate steps to maintain the confidentiality of participants. It is still unclear, however, whether the patients knowingly and willingly participated in the research. Nursing home residents are a vulnerable group. They may not have been aware of their right to refuse to be interviewed without fear of repercussion. Godine could have enhanced the ethical aspects of the study by taking more vigorous steps to obtain the informed, voluntary consent of the nursing home residents or to exclude patients who could not reasonably be expected to understand the researcher's request. Given the vulnerability of the group, Godine might also have established her own review panel composed of peers and interested lay people to review the ethical dimensions of her project. Debriefing sessions with study participants would also have been appropriate.*

2. Here is a brief description of ethical aspects of another fictitious study. Read the description and then respond to the questions that follow.

   Portnoy (1996) investigated the behavior of nursing students in crisis or emergency situations. The investigator was interested in comparing the behaviors of students from baccalaureate versus diploma programs to determine the adequacy of the preparation given to students in handling emergencies. Fifty students from both types of programs volunteered to partici-

pate in the study. The investigator wanted to observe reactions to crises as they might occur naturally, so the participants were not told the exact nature of the study. Each student was instructed to take the vital signs of a "patient," purportedly to evaluate the students' skills. The "patient," who was described as another student but who in fact was a confederate of the investigator, simulated an epileptic seizure while the vital signs were being taken. A research assistant, who was unaware of the purpose of the study and who did not know the educational background of the subjects, observed the timeliness and appropriateness of the students' responses through a one-way mirror. Subjects were not required to divulge their identities. Immediately after participation, subjects were debriefed as to the true nature of the study and were paid a $10 stipend.

Consider the aspects of this study with regard to the issues discussed in this chapter. To assist in your review, you can answer the questions below, as well as the questions in Box 5-2 of the textbook.

a. Were the subjects in this study at risk of physical or psychological harm? Were they at risk of exploitation?

b. Did the subjects in the study derive any benefits from their participation? Did the nursing community or society at large benefit? How would you assess the risk/benefit ratio?

c. Were the subjects' rights to self-determination violated? Was there any coercion involved? Was full disclosure made to subjects before participation? Was informed consent given to subjects and documented?

d. Were subjects treated fairly? Was their right to privacy protected?

e. What ethical dilemmas does this study present? How, if at all, can the dilemmas be resolved? To what extent *were* they resolved?

f. What type of human subjects review would be appropriate for a study such as the one described?

3. Read one or more of the articles listed below. Respond to parts a to f of Question D.2 (as well as questions from Box 5-2 of the textbook) in terms of these actual research studies.

- Chalmers, K., & Thomson, K. (1996). Coming to terms with the risk of breast cancer: Perception of women with primary relatives with breast cancer. *Qualitative Health Research, 6,* 256–282.

- Douglass, S., Daley, B. J., Rudy, E. B., Sereika, S. M., Menzel, L., Song, R., Dyer, M. A., & Montenegro, H. D. (1996). Survival experience of chronically critically ill patients. *Nursing Research, 45,* 73–77.

- Fuller, B. F., & Connor, D. A. (1996). Distribution of cues across assessed levels of infant pain. *Clinical Nursing Research, 5,* 167–184.

■ Woods, N. F., & Mitchell, E. S. (1996). Patterns of depressed mood in midlife women: Observations from the Seattle midlife women's health study. *Research in Nursing and Health, 19,* 111–123.

▨ E. SPECIAL PROJECTS

1. Prepare a brief summary of a hypothetical study in which the costs and benefits were both high. When the costs and benefits are essentially balanced, how should the researcher decide whether to proceed?

2. Skim the following research report, and draft an informed consent form for this study.

■ Mullins, I. L. (1996). Nurse caring behaviors for persons with acquired immunodeficiency syndrome/human immunodeficiency virus. *Applied Nursing Research, 9,* 18–23.

Designs for Nursing Research

PART III

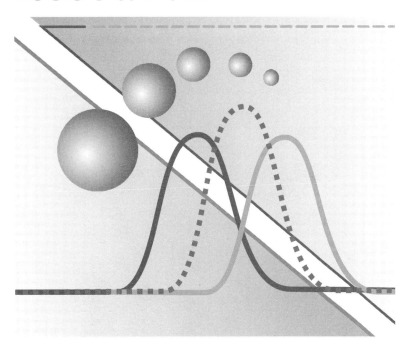

Chapter 6
Research Design for Quantitative Studies

◩ A. MATCHING EXERCISES

1. Match each research question from Set B with one (or more) of the phrases from Set A that indicates a potential reason for using a nonexperimental design. Indicate the letter(s) corresponding to your response next to each statement in Set B.

Set A

a. Independent variable cannot be manipulated
b. Ethical constraints on manipulation
c. Practical constraints on manipulation
d. No constraints on manipulation

Set B   *Responses*

1. Does the use of certain tampons cause toxic shock syndrome?   _____
2. Does heroin addiction among mothers affect the Apgar scores
   of their infants?   _____
3. Is the age of a hemodialysis patient related to the incidence
   of the disequilibrium syndrome?   _____
4. What body positions aid respiratory function?   _____
5. Does the ingestion of saccharin cause cancer in humans?   _____
6. Is a nurse's attitude toward the elderly related to his or her
   choice of a clinical specialty?   _____
7. Does the use of touch by nursing staff affect patient morale?   _____
8. Does a nurse's gender affect his or her salary and rate of
   promotion?   _____
9. Does extreme athletic exertion in young women cause
   amenorrhea?   _____
10. Does assertiveness training affect a psychiatric nurse's job
    performance?   _____

2. Match each problem statement from Set B with one (or more) of the types of research listed in Set A. Indicate the letter(s) corresponding to your response next to each of the statements in Set B.

Set A

a. Survey research
b. Evaluation research
c. Methodologic research
d. Needs assessment

Set B

Responses

1. What types of social and health service are needed by the rural elderly? _____

2. Does the assurance of anonymity to respondents increase self-reports of socially undesirable behavior, such as child or spouse abuse? _____

3. Do parents approve of sex education in the schools? _____

4. Does an intervention designed to provoke laughter reduce anxiety in hospitalized children? _____

5. What type of health services would best serve the homeless? _____

6. Is a radio-based media campaign more effective than a print-based media campaign in recruiting blood donors? _____

7. How does the general public feel about euthanasia? _____

8. Does the block-rotation method of scheduling result in a lower absentee rate among nursing staff than a random rotation method? _____

◪ B. COMPLETION EXERCISES

Write the words or phrases that correctly complete the sentences below.

1. The aspect of quantitative research design that concerns whether there is an intervention involves the distinction between _____ and _____ designs.

2. Quantitative researchers generally design their studies to include one or more types of _____.

3. In an experiment, the researcher manipulates the _____ variable.

4. The manipulation that the researcher introduces is referred to as the experimental _____.

5. Randomization is performed so that groups will be formed without _____ _____.

6. When data are gathered before the institution of some treatment, the initial data gathering is referred to as the _____.

7. When more than one independent variable is being simultaneously manipulated by the researcher, the design is referred to as a(n) _____.

8. Each factor in an experimental design must have two or more _____ _____.

9. When neither the subjects nor the individuals collecting data know in which group a subject is participating, the procedures are called _____ _____.

10. Subjects serve as their own controls in a(n) _____ _____ design.

11. A primary objective of a true experiment is to enable the researcher to infer _____.

12. When a true experimental design is not used, the control group is usually referred to as the _____ group.

13. A research design that involves a manipulation but lacks the controls of a quasi-experiment is referred to as a(n) _____ design.

14. A quasi-experimental design that involves repeated observations over time is referred to as a(n) _____ design.

15. The difficulty with a nonequivalent control group design is that the experimental and comparison groups cannot be assumed to be _____ before the intervention.

16. When no variable is manipulated in a study, the research is called _____.

17. In ex post facto research, the investigator forfeits control over the _____ variable.

18. In ex post facto research, it is difficult, if not impossible, to establish _____ relationships.

19. A prospective design is more rigorous in elucidating causal relations than a _____ design.

20. When data are collected at more than one point in time, the design is referred to as _____.

21. Longitudinal studies conducted to determine the long-term outcomes of some condition or intervention are called _____.

22. The type of study that collects extensive self-report information on people's attitudes, actions, beliefs, and intentions is called _____.

23. The effectiveness of a policy or program is studied in a(n) _____ .

24. The method of collecting needs assessment data by questioning knowledgeable people is known as the _____ approach.

25. Methodologic research is research conducted for the purpose of developing or refining research _____.

26. The environment should be controlled by the researcher insofar as possible by maximizing _____ in research conditions.

27. Using the principle of homogeneity to control extraneous variables limits the _____ of the findings.

28. Control over extraneous variables is required for the _____ validity of the study.

29. The differential loss of subjects from comparison groups is the threat known as _____.

30. Changes that occur as the result of time passing rather than as a result of the effects of the independent variable represent the threat of _____.

▨ C. STUDY QUESTIONS

1. Define the following terms. Use the textbook to compare your definition with the definition in Chapter 6 or in the Glossary.

   a. Research design: _____

   b. Extraneous variable: _____

   c. Manipulation: _____

   d. Randomization: _____

   e. Control group: _____

   f. Interaction effects: _____

   g. Clinical trial: _____

   h. Hawthorne effect: _____

   i. Quasi-experimental design: _____

j. Ex post facto research: _____

_____

k. Retrospective study: _____

_____

l. Prospective study: _____

_____

m. Case control study: _____

_____

n. Cross-sectional study: _____

_____

o. Trend study: _____

_____

p. Panel study: _____

_____

q. Randomized block design: _____

_____

r. Matching: _____

_____

s. Internal validity: _____

_____

t. Selection threat: _____

_____

u. Attrition: _____

_____

v. External validity: _____

_____

2. Which of the following variables are *inherently* not amenable to research manipulation*?

	Can Be Manipulated	*Cannot Be Manipulated*
a. Age at onset of obesity	_____	_____
b. Amount of auditory stimulation	_____	_____
c. Number of cigarettes smoked	_____	_____

Manipulation does not mean that the variable can be *affected* by a researcher; it refers to the researcher's ability to randomly assign people to different levels of the variable or to different groups.

    d. Infant's birth weight   _____   _____

    e. Blood type   _____   _____

    f. Preoperative anxiety   _____   _____

    g. Amount and timing of endotracheal suctioning   _____   _____

    h. Attitudes toward abortion   _____   _____

    i. Nurses' shift assignment   _____   _____

    j. Method of birth control used   _____   _____

    k. Mother–infant bonding   _____   _____

    l. Use of A-V shunt versus A-V fistula   _____   _____

    m. Amount of fluid intake   _____   _____

    n. Morale of AIDS patients   _____   _____

    o. Frequency of turning patients   _____   _____

3. A nurse researcher found a relationship between teenagers' level of knowledge about birth control and their level of sexual activity. That is, teenagers with higher levels of sexual activity knew more about birth control than teenagers with less sexual activity. Suggest at least three interpretations for this finding:

    a. _____

    _____

    _____

    b. _____

    _____

    _____

    c. _____

    _____

    _____

Does this research situation describe a research problem that is *inherently* nonexperimental? Why or why not?

4. A researcher found that supervisors' ratings of nurses' job performance were related to the nurses' self-reported job satisfaction. That is, nurses who received better job evaluations were more satisfied with their jobs than nurses with lower ratings. Suggest at least three interpretations for this result.

a. _____

_____

_____

b. _____

_____

_____

c. _____

_____

_____

Does this research situation describe a research problem that is *inherently* nonexperimental? Why or why not?

5. Refer to the 10 hypotheses in Questions C.4 and C.5 of Chapter 3. Indicate below whether these hypotheses could be tested using an experimental or quasi-experimental approach, a nonexperimental approach, or both.

Experimental or Quasi-Experimental	*Nonexperimental*	*Both*
4a. _____	_____	_____
4b. _____	_____	_____
4c. _____	_____	_____
4d. _____	_____	_____
4e. _____	_____	_____
5a. _____	_____	_____
5b. _____	_____	_____
5c. _____	_____	_____
5d. _____	_____	_____
5e. _____	_____	_____

6. Examine the 10 research questions in the first matching exercise of this chapter. For each, specify one or more extraneous variables that the researcher might want to control.

1. _____

2. _____

3. _____

    4. _____

    5. _____

    6. _____

    7. _____

    8. _____

    9. _____

  10. _____

7. A nurse researcher is interested in comparing the oral and rectal temperature measurements of febrile adults two times a day on three different wards. Could such a study be conducted as a factorial experiment? Why or why not? If yes, what are the factors in the design? Could a randomized block design be used? Why or why not? If yes, what would the blocking variable(s) be?

8. Suppose you wanted to evaluate the effect of an experimental approach to teaching student nurses how to give subcutaneous injections. In conducting a true experiment for this study, what environmental factors would you want to control to maintain the constancy of research conditions?

9. Below are several research problems. Indicate for each whether you think the problem should be studied using a survey approach or using an in-depth qualitative approach. Justify your response.

  a. By what process do new nursing home residents learn to adapt to their environments?

    _____

    _____

  b. To what extent are dietary habits and exercise patterns in healthy adults related?

    _____

    _____

c. What is the relationship between a teenager's health-risk appraisal and various forms of risk-taking behavior (e.g., smoking, sexual activity without contraception, using drugs, and so forth)?

_____

_____

d. What aspects of the lifestyles of urban disadvantaged women place them at especially high risk of pregnancy and childbirth complications?

_____

_____

e. How are the dynamics of nurse–patient interaction affected by the presence of a physician?

_____

_____

10. In the following study, the researchers conducted a double-blind experiment. Review the design for the study, and comment on the appropriateness of the double-blind procedures. What biases were the researchers trying to avoid? Were they successful?

- Simms, S. G., Rhodes, V. A., & Madsen, R. W. (1993). Comparison of prochlorperazine and lorazepam antiemetic regimens in the control of postchemotherapy symptoms. _Nursing Research, 42,_ 234–239.

▨ D. APPLICATION EXERCISES

1. Below is a brief description of the research design for a fictitious study, followed by a critique. Do you agree with the critique? Can you add other comments relevant to the research design of this study? (Box 6-1 offers some guiding questions.)

> ***Fictitious Study.*** *Bikowicz (1997) hypothesized that nursing effectiveness is higher in primary nursing than in team nursing. To test this hypothesis, she obtained data based on the nursing care of 100 patients in two medical-surgical units at the Wilton Hospital (which used primary nursing) and data from a similar sample of patients hospitalized at Ballston Hospital (which used team nursing). In both cases, the nursing*

approach was one that had been in place for more than 5 years. Bikowicz used three measures of nursing effectiveness: patients' length of stay in hospital; ratings of effectiveness by an objective expert observer; and total number of errors of omission and commission by the nursing staff. Bikowicz realized that numerous factors influence nursing effectiveness and that these factors needed to be controlled to test the research hypothesis. However, random assignment of nurses to the two types of nursing and random assignment of patients to hospitals was not possible. Therefore, Bikowicz took other steps to enhance the internal validity of the study. First, she designed her study in such a way that the conditions in the two hospitals were as comparable as possible. For example, she selected two private hospitals that were similar in size, modernity, reputation, nurses' pay scale, and proximity to an urban center. She focused on two medical–surgical units that were similar with respect to staff–patient ratio, number of beds, type of medical problems, and number of private and semiprivate rooms.

Bikowicz also recognized that staff characteristics were important. Therefore, a group of 25 nurses in each hospital who provided the care during the study were matched with respect to number of years of nursing experience (more than 5 years or fewer than 5 years) and educational credentials (baccalaureate degree or not). Finally, the 100 patients in each hospital were matched in terms of their gender and age (in 5-year groupings).

The data were collected by two objective observers who had no affiliation with either of the two hospitals and no personal acquaintance with any of the nursing staff or patients. The data supported Bikowicz's hypothesis that primary nursing is more effective than team nursing.

***Critique.** Bikowicz was interested in elucidating a causal relationship between type of nursing and nursing effectiveness; in essence, she was performing an evaluation of nursing approach. Given this aim, her decision to design a tightly controlled study seems well advised, particularly given the nonexperimental nature of the study. Bikowicz had no control over the implementation of either the primary or the team nursing. She tested her hypothesis using intact, preestablished groups of nurses and their patients.[†]*

[†]If Bikowicz had done the study at the time the hospital instituted the primary nursing approach (*i.e.,* if the study was part of the implementation process), the design would be considered quasi-experimental.

Although Bikowicz had to work with existing conditions, she nevertheless was careful in designing a study that controlled for numerous external and intrinsic extraneous variables. She maintained constancy over numerous external conditions, such as the hospital settings and the data collection procedures.

Bikowicz controlled several important intrinsic characteristics (of both nurses and patients) through matching. Although this procedure has numerous shortcomings, the use of matching was in this case preferable to totally ignoring the problem of extraneous variables. One alternative would have been to use the principle of homogeneity (e.g., use all baccalaureate nurses with more than 5 years of experience, or use patients in a similar age range), but this would have severely limited the generalizability of the results. The problem with matching, as noted earlier, is that only two or three matching variables can be used, and there may be far more than two or three extraneous variables. For example, such factors as a nurse's age, amount of continuing education, level of empathy, and attitudes toward type of nursing approach presumably affect nursing effectiveness. If systematic differences in these variables exist between nurses in the two hospitals (or if there were other important differences between the two groups of patients), then such differences represent rival explanations, competing with the type of nursing approach as causes of the differences in the ratings of nursing effectiveness. Thus, selection is the primary threat to the internal validity of this study. If some external event affecting nursing performance occurred in one or both hospitals during the data collection period, then history might also have been a threat.

In summary, the researcher took many commendable steps to control extraneous variables in this study. Given the constraints of not being able to manipulate the independent variable (i.e., randomize nurses and patients to groups or randomize hospitals to type of nursing approach), matching was one of the best alternatives for controlling extraneous variables. The only more rigorous approach would have been to gather data on any other extraneous variables (e.g., nurses' ages or amounts of continuing education) and to control these variables statistically using analysis of covariance. It might be noted that Bikowicz might have strengthened her conclusions regarding the effectiveness of primary versus team nursing if she had undertaken in-depth case studies of the nursing care of typical patients in both hospitals.

2. Here is a brief summary of another fictitious study. Read the summary and then respond to the questions that follow.

> *DeSeve (1996) wanted to test the effectiveness of a new relaxation and biofeedback intervention on menopause symptoms. She invited women who presented themselves in an outpatient clinic with complaints of severe hot flashes to participate in the study of the experimental treatment. These 30 women were asked to record, every day for 1 week before their treatment, the frequency and duration of their hot flashes. During the intervention, which involved six 1-hour sessions over a 3-week period, the women again recorded their symptoms. Then, 4 weeks after the treatment, the women were asked to record their hot flashes over a 5-day period. At the end of the study, DeSeve found that both the frequency and average duration of the hot flashes had been significantly reduced in this sample of women. She concluded that her new treatment was an effective alternative to estrogen replacement therapy in treating menopausal hot flashes.*

Review and critique this study. Suggest alternative designs for testing the effectiveness of the treatment. To assist you in your critique, here are some guiding questions. (See also the critiquing guidelines in Box 6-1 of the textbook.)

a. Is the design of this study experimental, quasi-experimental, preexperimental, or nonexperimental?

b. Evaluate the internal validity of the study. Does the design eliminate or minimize the threat of history? selection? maturation? mortality?

c. The investigator concluded that the outcome (*i.e.*, the reduction in the frequency and duration of the women's hot flashes) was attributable to the treatment. Can you offer one or more alternative explanations to account for the outcome?

d. Consider your responses to parts **b** and **c** above. If you have identified any weaknesses in the design of this research, suggest a modified design that would improve the internal validity of the study. In what way does your new design eliminate the problems of the original design? Have you dealt with all of the threats to the study's internal validity?

e. Does this study fall into a category described in the section of the chapter on additional types of research (*i.e.*, is it a survey, needs assessment, etc.)?

3. Below are several suggested research articles. Read the introductory and methods sections of one or more of these articles and respond to parts **a** to **e** from Question D.2 in terms of these actual research studies.

- Grant, L. P., Wagner, L. I., & Neill, K. M. (1994). Fiber-fortified feedings in immobile patients. *Clinical Nursing Research, 3,* 166–172.

- Ganong, L. H. & Coleman, M. (1992). The effect of clients' family structure on nursing students' cognitive schemas and verbal behavior. *Research in Nursing & Health, 15,* 139–146.
- Roberts, B. L., & Palmer, R. (1996). Cardiac response of elderly adults to normal activities and aerobic walking. *Clinical Nursing Research, 5,* 105–115.
- Oertwich, P. A., Kindschuh, A. M., & Bergstrom, N. (1995). The effects of small shifts in body weight on blood flow and interface pressure. *Research in Nursing and Health, 18,* 481–488.
- Schilke, J. M., Johnson, G. O., Housh, T. J., & O'Dell, J. R. (1996). Effects of muscle-strength training on the functional status of patients with osteoarthritis of the knee joint. *Nursing Research, 45,* 68–71.

4. Another brief summary of a fictitious study follows. Read the summary and then respond to the questions that follow.

Auclair (1996) hypothesized that the absence of socioemotional supports among the elderly results in a high level of chronic health problems and low morale. She tested this hypothesis by interviewing a sample of 250 residents of one community who were aged 65 years and older. The respondents were randomly selected from a list of town residents. Auclair used several measures of the availability of socioemotional supports: (1) whether the respondent lived with any kin; (2) whether the respondent had any living children who resided within 30 minutes away; (3) the total number of interactions the respondent had had in the previous week with kin not residing in his or her household; and (4) the number of close friends in whom the respondent thought he or she could confide. Based on responses to the various questions on social support, respondents were classified in one of three groups: low social support, moderate social support, and high social support. In a 6-month follow-up interview, Auclair collected information from 214 respondents about the frequency and intensity of the respondents' illnesses in the preceding 6 months, their hospitalization records, their overall satisfaction with life, and their attitudes toward their own aging. An analysis of the data showed that the low-support group had significantly more health problems, lower life satisfaction ratings, and lower acceptance of their aging than the other two groups. Auclair concluded that the availability of social supports resulted in better physical and mental adjustment to old age.

Review and critique this study. Suggest alternative designs for testing the researcher's hypotheses. To assist you in your critique, here are some guiding questions. (See also the critiquing guidelines in Box 6-1 of the textbook.)

a. Is the design described above experimental, quasi-experimental, preexperimental, or nonexperimental? If it is nonexperimental, is it inherently so? Why or why not?

b. Evaluate the internal validity of the study. What threats to its internal validity, if any, are posed?

c. Examine the criteria for causality presented in Chapter 6 of the textbook. Does this study meet all the criteria for establishing causality?

d. The researcher concluded that her independent variable (amount of social support) "caused" certain outcomes (mental and physical health status in the elderly). Can you offer two or more alternative explanations to account for the findings?

e. Consider your responses to parts **b** through **d** above. If you have identified any weaknesses in the design of the research, suggest modifications that would improve the internal validity of the study.

f. Does this study fall into a category described in the section of the chapter on additional types of research (*i.e.*, is it a survey, evaluation, etc.)?

5. Below are several suggested research articles. Read the introductory and methods sections of one or more of these articles and respond to parts a to f of Question D.4 above in terms of these actual research studies.

- Broom, B. L. (1994). Impact of marital quality and psychological well-being on parental sensitivity. *Nursing Research, 43,* 138–143.
- Hill, P. D., & Aldag, J. C. (1996). Smoking and breastfeeding status. *Research in Nursing and Health, 19,* 125–132.
- Horns, P. N., Ratcliffe, L. P., Leggett, J. C., & Swanson, M. S. (1996). Pregnancy outcomes among active and sedentary primiparous women. *Journal of Obstetric, Gynecologic, and Neonatal Nursing, 25,* 49–54.
- McFarlane, J., & Parker, B. (1996). Physical abuse, smoking, and substance use during pregnancy: Prevalence, interrelationships, and effects on birth weight. *Journal of Obstetric, Gynecologic, and Neonatal Nursing, 25,* 313–320.

6. Another brief summary of the research design for a fictitious study follows. Read the summary and then answer the questions that follow.

Neudel (1997) investigated the relationship between the use of intrauterine devices (IUDs) and the incidence of pelvic inflammatory disease (PID) in a sample of urban women. The data were gathered from the gynecology departments of four health centers (one university, one city hospital, one health maintenance organization, and one consortium of private gynecologists). Neudel obtained the records of 600 women—150 from each facility—who were diagnosed within the previous

*12 months as having PID. She also obtained the records of 150
women who had come to each of the facilities for some other
purpose and who had no record of having had PID within the
12-month period before their focal visit. The two groups of 600
women (the PID and non-PID group) were matched in terms
of age (within 5-year ranges of 20 or younger, 21 to 25, 26 to
30, 31 to 35 years old, etc.) and marital status (currently married or not married). For each of the 1200 women, the records
were examined to determine whether they had had an IUD
inserted within 2 years before their focal visit. For those
women for whom no determination could be made based
on the records of the facility, brief telephone interviews were
administered to obtain the needed information (30 women
who could not be reached were replaced with other women
to maintain the sample size). The data showed that 122
women in the PID group (20.3%), compared with 74 women
in the non-PID group (12.3%), had used an IUD, a significant
group difference. Based on this analysis, Neudel concluded
that use of an IUD was a causative factor of PID in this
sample.*

Review and critique this study. Suggest alternative designs for testing the researcher's hypotheses. To assist you in your critique, here are some guiding
questions. (See also the critiquing guidelines in Box 6-1 of the textbook.)

a. Apply parts a through e of Question D.4 to this current example.
b. What extraneous variables did the researcher identify, and by what method
were they controlled? How else might they have been controlled?
c. What extraneous variables do you think *should* have been controlled but
were not? Why might the researcher have decided not to control these variables?
d. To what extent did the researcher control for the constancy of conditions
in this study? Suggest ways in which this aspect of the study could have
been improved.
e. Evaluate the external validity of the study in terms of the threats described
in Chapter 6 of the textbook. What changes, if any, would you recommend
to improve the external validity of the design?
f. Does this study fall into a category described in the section of the chapter
on additional types of research (*i.e.*, is it a survey, needs assessment, etc.)?

7. Below are several suggested research articles. Read the introductory and
methods sections of one or more of these articles and respond to parts a to f of
Question D.6 in terms of these actual research studies.

- Esparza, D. V., & Esperat, M. C. R. (1996). The effects of childhood sexual
abuse on minority adolescent mothers. *Journal of Obstetric, Gynecologic,
and Neonatal Nursing, 25,* 321–328.

- Gross, D., Fogg, L., & Tucker, S. (1995). The efficacy of parent training for promoting positive parent-toddler relationships. *Research in Nursing and Health, 18,* 489–499.
- Hahn, W. K., Brooks, J. A., & Hartsough, D. M. (1993). Self-disclosure and coping styles in men with cardiovascular reactivity. *Research in Nursing and Health, 16,* 275–282.
- Tumulty, G., Jernigan, I. E., & Kohut, G. F. (1994). The impact of perceived work environment on job satisfaction of hospital staff. *Applied Nursing Research, 7,* 84–90.

8. Below is another description of the research design for a fictitious study. Read the summary and then respond to the questions that follow.

Poole (1996) hypothesized that aging negatively affects intellectual capacity and motor responsivity. To test this hypothesis, she randomly selected the names of 250 men aged 70 years or older, 250 men in their 50s, and 250 men in their 30s from the residents living in a mid-sized city in Illinois. Poole realized that intellectual capacity is sometimes correlated with social class. Furthermore, mortality rates vary by social class. Therefore, the subjects were selected in such a way that half in each group were from lower-income households (household income $20,000 or less) and half were from higher-income households (income over $20,000). The basic design for the analysis, therefore, was as follows:

	Age Group		
Income	30s	50s	70s
≤ $20,000			
> $20,000			

The 750 people were administered an intelligence test that measured verbal aptitude, problem solving, quantitative skills, spatial aptitude, and overall intelligence. In addition, the subjects were given various reaction-time tests. The analysis of the data showed that, as hypothesized, intelligence declined with age in both income groups. Except on the measure of verbal aptitude, the subjects in their 30s scored highest, and the subjects in their 70s scored lowest on the subtests of intellectual capacity and on overall intelligence. The same pattern was observed for reaction time. Poole concluded that the aging process causes deterioration of both intellectual and motor capacity.

Review and critique Poole's study. Suggest alternative designs or other modifications for testing the researcher's hypothesis. Use parts a through e from Question D.6 to guide you in your critique. In addition, answer the following questions:

a. Is this design cross-sectional or longitudinal?

b. What problems, if any, does this design pose in terms of testing the hypothesis?

c. What design, if any, might be more appropriate?

d. What difficulties, if any, would Poole have had in implementing your recommended design?

e. Does this study fall into a category described in the section of the chapter on additional types of research (*i.e.,* is it a survey, field study, etc.)?

9. Below are several suggested research articles. Read the introductory and methods sections of one or more of these articles and respond to parts a through e of Question D.8 in terms of these actual research studies.

■ Beach, E. K., Maloney, B. H., Plocica, A. R., Sherry, S. E., Weaver, M., Luthringer, L., & Utz, S. (1992). The spouse: A factor in recovery after acute myocardial infarction. *Heart and Lung, 21,* 30–38.

■ Heidrich, S. M. (1993). The relationship between physical health and psychological well-being in elderly women: A developmental perspective. *Research in Nursing and Health, 16,* 123–130.

■ Polivka, B. J., Nickel, J. T., & Wilkins, J. R. (1993). Cerebral palsy: Evaluation of a model of risk. *Research in Nursing and Health, 16*(3), 113–122.

■ Walker, L. O. & Montgomery, E. (1994). Maternal identity and role attainment: Long-term relations to children's development. *Nursing Research, 43,* 105–110.

■ Youngblut, J. M. (1995). Consistency between maternal employment attitudes and employment status. *Research in Nursing and Health, 18,* 501–513.

▧ E. SPECIAL PROJECTS

1. Suppose that you were interested in testing the hypothesis that a regular regimen of exercise reduces blood pressure, improves cardiovascular efficiency, and increases coronary circulation. Design a quasi-experiment to test the hypothesis. Evaluate the design with regard to its internal validity. Design a true experiment to test the same hypothesis and compare the internal validity of this design with that of the quasi-experiment. What are the most salient threats to the internal validity of the two designs?

2. Suppose that you were interested in testing the hypothesis that the use of oral contraceptives caused breast cancer. Describe how such a hypothesis could be tested using a retrospective design. Now describe a prospective design for the same study. Compare the strengths and weaknesses of the two approaches. Could an experimental or quasi-experimental design be used? Why or why not?

3. Suppose that you wanted to compare premature and normal infants in terms of their development at age 5. Describe how you would design such a study, being careful to indicate what extraneous variables you would need to control and how you would control them.

4. Suppose that you were interested in studying short-term versus long-term impacts of the death of a spouse on the physical and mental health of the surviving spouse. Design a cross-sectional study to research the question, specifying the characteristics of your sample. Now design a longitudinal study for the same problem. Identify the advantages and disadvantages of the two designs.

Chapter 7
Qualitative Research Design and Approaches

▨ A. MATCHING EXERCISES

1. Match each descriptive statement from Set B with one of the research traditions from Set A. Indicate the letter corresponding to your response next to each item in Set B.

Set A

a. Ethnography
b. Phenomenology
c. Grounded theory
d. Ethnography, phenomenology, and grounded theory

Set B   *Responses*

1. Is rooted in a philosophical tradition developed by Husserl and Heidegger   _____
2. Studies both broadly defined cultures and more narrowly defined ones   _____
3. Uses qualitative data to address questions of interest   _____
4. Is an approach to the study of social processes and social structures   _____
5. Is concerned with the lived experiences of humans   _____
6. Strives to achieve an emic perspective on the members of a group   _____
7. Is closely related to a research tradition called hermeneutics _____
8. Uses a procedure referred to as constant comparison   _____
9. Stems from a discipline other than nursing   _____
10. Developed by the sociologists Glaser and Strauss   _____

2. Match each descriptive statement from Set B with one of the statements from Set A. Indicate the letter corresponding to your response next to each item in Set B.

Set A

a. Qualitative studies
b. Quantitative studies
c. Both qualitative and quantitative studies
d. Neither qualitative nor quantitative studies

Set B   *Responses*

1. Should be undertaken to help improve nursing practice   _____
2. Are especially useful for understanding dynamic processes   _____
3. Can play a role in the development of new instruments   _____
4. Are useful in proving the validity of theories   _____
5. Can complement the strengths and weaknesses of the other approach   _____
6. Can sometimes be productively embedded within a survey   _____
7. Can contribute to theoretical insights   _____
8. Tend to involve small samples   _____

▨ B. COMPLETION EXERCISES

Write the words or phrases that correctly complete the sentences below.

1. The disciplinary root of ethnography is _____; of ethology is _____; and of ethnomethodology is _____.
2. Ethnographic research focuses on human _____.
3. The concept _____ is frequently used by ethnographers to describe the significant role of the researcher in interpreting a culture.
4. Phenomenologic research focuses on the _____ of phenomena as experienced by people.
5. Phenomenologists study the various aspects of the lived experience including lived space or _____; lived body or _____; lived time or _____; or lived human relations or _____.
6. The primary purpose of _____ is to generate comprehensive explanations of phenomena that are grounded in reality.
7. Qualitative and quantitative data are often _____ in that they mutually supply each other's lack.
8. A major advantage of integrating different approaches is potential enhancements to the study's _____.

◪ C. STUDY QUESTIONS

1. Define the following terms. Use the textbook to compare your definition with the definition in Chapter 7 or in the Glossary.

a. Discourse analyses: _____

_____

b. Hermeneutics: _____

_____

c. Historical research: _____

_____

d. Emic perspective: _____

_____

e. Etic perspective: _____

_____

f. Ethnonursing research: _____

_____

g. Being-in-the-world: _____

_____

h. Bracketing: _____

_____

i. Multimethod research: _____

_____

2. For each of the research questions below, indicate what type of research tradition would likely guide the inquiry.

a. What is the social psychological process experienced by couples experiencing infertility?

_____

_____

b. How does the culture of a suicide survivors self-help group facilitate the grieving process?

_____

_____

c. What are the power dynamics that arise in conversations between nurses and bed-ridden nursing home patients?

_____

_____

d. What is the lived experience of the spousal caretaker of an Alzheimer's patient?

_____

_____

3. Read one of the following studies, in which qualitative data were gathered and analyzed to address a research question. Suggest ways in which the collection of quantitative data might have enriched the study, strengthened its validity, or enhanced its interpretability.
   - Manfredi, C. M. (1996). A descriptive study of nurse managers and leadership. *Western Journal of Nursing Research, 18,* 314–329.
   - Milliken, P. J., & Northcott, H. C. (1996). Seeking validation: Hypothyroidism and the chronic illness trajectory. *Qualitative Health Research, 6,* 202–223.
   - Redfern-Vance, N. & Hutchinson, S. A. (1995). The process of developing personal sovereignty in women who repeatedly acquire sexually transmitted diseases. *Qualitative Health Research, 5,* 222–236.
   - Singer, N. (1995). Understanding sexual risk behavior from drug users' accounts of their life experiences. *Qualitative Health Research, 5,* 237–249.
4. Read one of the following studies in which quantitative data were gathered and analyzed to address a research question. Suggest ways in which the collection of qualitative data might have enriched the study, strengthened its validity, or enhanced its interpretability.
   - Bailey, B. J. (1996). Mediators of depression in adults with diabetes. *Clinical Nursing Research, 5,* 28–42.
   - Birenbaum, L. K., Stewart, B.J., & Phillips, D. S. (1996). Health status of bereaved parents. *Nursing Research, 45,* 105–109.
   - Goldstein, N. L., Snyder, M., Edin, C., Lindgren, B., & Finkelstein, S. M. (1996). Comparison of two teaching strategies. *Clinical Nursing Research, 5,* 150–166.
   - Nickel, J. T., Salsberry, P. J., Caswell, R. J., Keller, M. D., Long, T., & O'Connell, M. (1996). Quality of life in nurse case management of persons with AIDS receiving home care. *Research in Nursing & Health, 19,* 91–99.

▨ D. APPLICATION EXERCISES

1. Below is a brief description of an integrated qualitative-quantitative study, followed by a critique. Do you agree with this critique? Can you add other comments regarding this study design? (Box 7-1 offers some guiding questions.)

   Fictitious Study. *Bristol (1996) conducted a study designed to examine the emotional well-being of women who had a mastectomy. Bristol wanted to develop an in-depth understanding of the emotional experiences of women as they recov-*

ered from their surgery, including the process by which they handled their fears, their concerns about their sexuality, their levels of anxiety and depression, their methods of coping, and their social supports.

Bristol's basic study design was a field study, loosely within a grounded theory tradition. She gathered information from a sample of 25 women, primarily by means of in-depth interviews with the women on two occasions. The first interviews were scheduled within 1 month after the surgery. Follow-up interviews were conducted about 12 months after the surgery. Several of the women in the sample participated in a support group, and Bristol attended and made observations at several of those meetings. Additionally, Bristol decided to interview the "significant other" (usually the women's husbands) of most of the women, when she learned that the women's emotional well-being was linked to the manner in which the significant other was reacting to the surgery.

In addition to the rich, in-depth information she gathered, Bristol wanted to be able to better interpret the emotional status of the women. Therefore, at both the original and follow-up interview with the women, she administered a psychological scale known as the Center for Epidemiological Studies Depression Scale (CES-D), a quantitative measure that has scores that can range from 0 to 60. This scale has been widely used in community populations, and has "cut-off" scores designating when a person is at risk of clinical depression (i.e., a score of 16 and above).

Bristol's qualitative analysis showed that the basic process underlying psychological recovery from the mastectomy was something she labeled "Gaining by Losing," a process that involved heightened self-awareness and self-respect after an initial period of despair and self-pity. The process also involved, for some, a strengthening of personal relationships with significant others, whereas for others, it resulted in the birth of awareness of fundamental deficiencies in their relationships. The quantitative findings confirmed that a very high percentage of women were at risk of being depressed at 1 month after the mastectomy, but at 12 months, levels of depression were actually modestly lower than in the general population of women.

Critique. *In her study, Bristol embedded a quantitative measure into the field work in an interesting manner. The bulk of data were qualitative—in-depth interviews and in-depth observations. However, she also opted to include a well-*

known measure of depression, which provides her with an important context for interpreting her data. A major advantage of using the CES-D (aside from the fact that the CES-D has a good reputation) is that this scale has known characteristics in the general population, and therefore provided a built-in "comparison group."

Bristol used a flexible design that allowed her to use her initial data to guide her inquiry. For example, she decided to conduct in-depth interviews with significant others when she learned their importance to the women's process of emotional recovery. Bristol did do some advance planning, however, that provided loose guidance. For example, although her questioning undoubtedly evolved while in the field, she had the foresight to realize that to capture a process, she would need to collect data longitudinally. She also made the up-front decision to use the CES-D to supplement the in-depth interviews.

*In this study, the findings from the qualitative and quantitative portions of the study were complementary. Both portions of the study confirmed that the women initially had emotional "losses," but eventually they recovered and "gained" in terms of their emotional well-being and their self-awareness. This example illustrates how the validity of study findings can be enhanced by the blending of qualitative and quantitative data. If the qualitative data alone had been gathered, Bristol might not have gotten a good handle on the degree to which the women had actually "recovered" (*vis à vis *women who had never had a mastectomy). Conversely, if she had collected only the CES-D data, she would have had no insights into the process by which the recovery occurred.*

2. Here is a brief summary of another fictitious study. Read the summary and then respond to the questions that follow.

Clark (1997) conducted a study to investigate breastfeeding practices among teenaged mothers, who have been found in many studies to be less likely than older mothers to breastfeed. Using birth records from two large hospitals, Clark contacted 250 young women between the ages of 15 and 19 who had given birth in the previous year and invited them to participate in a survey. Those who agreed to participate (185 teenaged mothers) were interviewed by telephone (when possible), using a structured interview that asked about breastfeeding practices, attitudes toward motherhood, and conflicting demands with regard to breastfeeding, such as school attendance or employment. Several psychological measures (including measures of self-esteem and self-efficacy) were also

administered. Teenagers without a telephone were inter-
viewed in person in their own homes. All of the teenagers in-
terviewed at home were also interviewed in greater depth; the
in-depth questions focused on such areas as feelings about
breastfeeding, the decision-making process that led them to
decide whether to breastfeed, barriers to breastfeeding, and
intentions to breastfeed with any subsequent children. Clark
used the quantitative data to determine the characteristics as-
sociated with breastfeeding status and duration. The qualita-
tive data were used to interpret and validate the quantitative
findings.

Review and critique this study. Suggest alternative data collection and analysis
approaches. To assist you in your critique, here are some guiding questions.

a. Which of the aims of integration, if any, were served by this study?

b. What was the researcher's basic strategy for integration? How effective was
this strategy in addressing the aims of integration?

c. Suggest ways of altering the design of the study and the data collection approach to further promote integrative aims.

d. Would the study have been stronger if it had involved the collection of
quantitative data only? Qualitative data only? Why or why not?

3. Below are several suggested research articles of studies that used an integrated approach. Read one or more of these articles and respond to parts a to
d of Question D.2 in terms of these actual research studies.

- Gil, V. E. (1995). The new female condom: Attitudes and opinions of low-
income Puerto Rican women at risk for HIV/AIDS. *Qualitative Health Research, 5,* 178–203.

- Halm, M. A., Titler, M. G., Kleiber, C., Johnson, S. K., Montgomery, L. A.,
Craft, M. J., Buckwalter, K., Nicholson, A., & Megivern, L. (1993). Behav-
ioral responses of family members during critical illness. *Clinical Nursing
Research, 2,* 414–437.

- Lev, E. L. (1992). Patients' strategies for adapting to cancer treatment.
Western Journal of Nursing Research, 14, 595–612.

- Long, K. A., & Weinert, C. (1992). Descriptions and perceptions of health
among rural and urban adults with multiple sclerosis. *Research in Nursing and Health, 15,* 335–342.

▨ E. SPECIAL PROJECTS

1. Prepare three research questions that would be amenable to multimethod research.

2. For one of the research questions suggested in Exercise E.1, write a two- to
three-page description of the types of data that might be collected and how the
use of both qualitative and quantitative data would strengthen the study.

Chapter 8
Sampling Designs

▨ A. MATCHING EXERCISES

1. Match each type of sampling approach from Set B with one of the phrases from Set A. Indicate the letter corresponding to your response next to each of the statements in Set B.

Set A

a. Sampling approach for quantitative studies
b. Sampling approach for qualitative studies
c. Sampling approach for either quantitative or qualitative studies
d. Sampling approach for neither quantitative nor qualitative studies

Set B   *Responses*

1. Typical case sampling   _____
2. Purposive sampling   _____
3. Cluster sampling   _____
4. Intensity sampling   _____
5. Homogeneous sampling   _____
6. Snowball sampling   _____
7. Stratified random sampling   _____
8. Quota sampling   _____
9. Power sampling   _____
10. Theory-based sampling   _____

2. Match each statement from Set B with one of the phrases from Set A. Indicate the letter corresponding to your response next to each of the statements in Set B.

Set A

a. Probability sampling
b. Nonprobability sampling
c. Both probability and nonprobability sampling
d. Neither probability nor nonprobability sampling

Set B   *Responses*

1. Includes systematic sampling procedures   _____
2. Allows an estimation of the magnitude of sampling error   _____
3. Guarantees a representative sample   _____
4. Includes quota sampling   _____
5. Yields more accurate results when the samples are large   _____
6. Elements are selected by nonrandom methods   _____
7. Can be used with entire populations or with selected strata
   from the populations   _____
8. Is used to select populations   _____
9. Provides an equal chance of elements being selected   _____
10. Is required when the population is homogeneous   _____

◩ B. COMPLETION EXERCISES

Write the words or phrases that correctly complete the sentences below.

1. A(n) _____ is a subset of the elements that constitute the population.

2. The main criterion for evaluating a sample in a quantitative study is its _____ _____ of the population being studied.

3. A sample in a quantitative study would be considered _____ _____ if it systematically overrepresented or underrepresented a segment of the population.

4. If a population is completely _____ with respect to key attributes, then any sample is as good as any other.

5. Another term used for convenience sample is _____ _____.

6. Quota samples are essentially convenience samples from selected _____ _____ of the population.

7. Another term for a purposive sampling in a quantitative context is _____ _____ sampling; in a qualitative context, the terms _____ or _____ _____ sampling are sometimes used for purposive sampling.

8. The most basic type of probability sampling is referred to as _____ _____.

9. When disproportionate sampling is used, an adjustment procedure known as _____ is normally used to estimate population values.

10. Another term used to refer to cluster sampling is _____ _____ sampling.

11. In systematic samples, the distance between selected elements is referred to as the _____.

12. Differences between population values and sample values are referred to as _____.

13. If a quantitative researcher has confidence in his or her sampling design, the results of a study can reasonably be generalized to the _____ _____ population.

14. As the size of a sample _____, the probability of drawing a deviant sample diminishes.

15. If a researcher wanted to draw a systematic sample of 100 from a population of 3000, the sampling interval would be _____.

16. In a qualitative study, sampling decisions are often guided by the potential a data source had to be _____-rich.

17. In _____ sampling, the qualitative researcher deliberately reduces variation, whereas in _____ _____ sampling, the researcher purposefully selects cases with a wide range of variation on dimensions of interest.

18. _____ sampling involves selecting study participants to highlight the average situation.

▨ C. STUDY QUESTIONS

1. Define the following terms. Use the textbook to compare your definition with the definition in Chapter 8 or in the Glossary.

   a. Population: _____ _____

   b. Probability sampling: _____ _____

   c. Nonprobability sampling: _____ _____

   d. Stratum: _____ _____

   e. Snowball sampling: _____ _____

   f. Quota sampling: _____ _____

g. Purposive sampling: _____

_____

h. Sampling frame: _____

_____

i. Disproportionate sample: _____

_____

j. Cluster sampling: _____

_____

k. Systematic sampling: _____

_____

l. Power analysis: _____

_____

m. Response rate: _____

_____

n. Theoretical sampling: _____

_____

o. Data saturation: _____

_____

2. Identify the type of sampling design used in the following examples:

Type of Design

a. Thirty nursing faculty randomly sampled from a random selection of 10 nursing schools   _____

b. All of the nurses participating in a continuing education seminar   _____

c. A sample of 250 members randomly selected from a roster of ANA members   _____

d. Every 20th patient admitted to the emergency room in the month of June   _____

e. The first 20 male and the first 20 female patients admitted to the hospital with hypothermia   _____

f. Fifteen cancer patients with extremely high levels of depression and 15 cancer patients with extremely low levels of depression   _____

g. Twenty-five people whose family members had attempted suicide, most of whom were referred by other members already in the sample   _____

3. Suppose a researcher has decided to use a systematic sampling design for a research project. The known population size is 4400, and the sample size desired is 200. What is the sampling interval? If the first element selected is 112, what would be the second, third, and fourth elements to be selected?

4. Read the following article and identify what the successive clusters were in drawing the research sample: Yarcheski, A., & Mahan, N. E. (1985). The unification model in nursing. *Nursing Research, 34,* 120–125.

5. Suppose a researcher were interested in studying the smoking habits of nurses in a quantitative survey. Suggest a possible target and accessible population for a researcher working in your area. What strata might be identified by the researcher if quota sampling were used?

6. Suppose a qualitative researcher wanted to study the life quality of cancer survivors. Suggest what the researcher might do to obtain a maximum variation sample; a typical case sample; a homogeneous sample; and an extreme case sample.

◪ D. APPLICATION EXERCISES

1. Below is a brief description of the sampling plan of a fictitious study, followed by a critique. Do you agree with this critique? Can you add other comments relevant to the sampling plan of this study? (Box 8-1 offers some guiding questions.)

    Fictitious Study. *Labenski (1997) designed a quantitative study to investigate nurses' attitudes toward surrogate motherhood, test-tube babies, and other nontraditional reproductive options. She defined her target population as all RNs in the*

United States. She realized, however, that she did not have direct access to the entire population for selecting a sample. Therefore, she specified as her accessible population RNs in the state of Massachusetts. She contacted the directors of nursing in 12 hospitals chosen to represent urban and rural settings and public and private auspices and enlisted their cooperation. She asked these directors to distribute 30 questionnaires to random samples of RNs in the hospitals. The number of completed questionnaires obtained from 10 hospitals (the other two hospitals did not wish to participate) ranged from a low of 16 to a high of 28, for a total of 238 completed questionnaires.

Critique. The sampling design used by Labenski is a multistage design that combines both nonprobability and probability components. Labenski handpicked 12 hospitals that yielded, in her judgment, a good mix in terms of locations and auspices. The first stage of the design, therefore, can be described as purposive sampling. Labenski could have obtained a listing of all Massachusetts facilities and randomly chosen 12. With such a small sample of hospitals, however, it is conceivable that a skewed sample might have been obtained (e.g., no rural hospitals). If the location and auspices of the hospital are related to nurses' opinions about nontraditional routes to parenthood, then Labenski's approach makes some sense, although stratification could have been used to address this problem. One of the difficulties with this sampling plan is that we cannot be sure that Labenski did not inadvertently handpick hospitals with other characteristics that might affect or be related to nurses' attitudes.

The second stage of the sampling plan involved a probability component. Within each hospital, the nursing directors were asked to select a simple random sample of 30 RNs and to distribute questionnaires to this group. Such a procedure presumably guaranteed that systematic biases would be minimized. Still, Labenski cannot be sure that biases were not introduced because she herself did not control the random selection. By allowing the directors of nursing to select the sample, the investigator risked (1) the directors' misunderstanding of how to select a random sample and (2) the directors' failing to comply with the request for random selection for some reason, such as practicality or personal considerations. For example, the director might decide to exclude Ms. Pehl from the sample because of a recent death in her family. By allowing others to perform the random selection, Labenski did not exercise as much control over the research situation as she might have. Furthermore, she risked additional bias stemming from low response rates in some hospitals (as low as 53% in one hospital). A personal delivery of the questionnaires and good follow-up procedures might have yielded a higher rate of returned questionnaires. Whenever response rates are low, there always remains the possibility of distortions because nonrespondents are rarely a random subsample of all possible subjects. For example, nonrespondents may be people with strong views on the issues in the questionnaire.

The key question that needs to be asked in evaluating a sampling design in a quantitative study is the following: Is the sample sufficiently representative of the population that the results can be generalized to that population? In Labenski's case, it would be unwise to conclude that the opinions of the 238 nurses surveyed could be generalized to all RNs in the United States, or even to all RNs in Massachusetts. Given Labenski's sampling plan, many nurses would never have had an opportunity to express their opinions. For example, unemployed nurses and RNs working in schools, community health centers, colleges, or businesses were not sampled, and their opinions might differ systematically from those working in Massachusetts hospitals. Furthermore, two hospitals refused to participate in the study, and in those that did cooperate, response rates were not high, yielding a relatively small sample size for a survey of this type.

Despite the fact that Labenski's sampling plan has some limitations, it is not without merit. She did well not to rely on a single hospital from which to collect data. Furthermore, gross distortions were undoubtedly avoided by requesting nursing directors to select a random sample of nurses rather than by simply handing out questionnaires to the first 30 nurses available. Labenski's results would have been enhanced had she exercised more control over sample selection and response rates, but they are nevertheless worthy of consideration. Part of the problem with the design is Labenski's definition of the population. If Labenski had specified a more modest target population (e.g., RNs currently employed in hospital settings in the northeast), then her sampling plan would have had more credibility.

2. Here is a brief summary of another fictitious study. Read the summary and then respond to the questions that follow.

   Dresser (1996) studied the job-search strategies of recent nursing school graduates. Her survey focused on such issues as timing of job applications, number of applications, source of information about jobs, method of initial contact, and so on. She was interested in learning whether certain strategies were more successful in achieving job offers than others. She obtained lists of graduates from six schools of nursing in the Washington, DC, area (two schools for each of three different types of programs). She then conducted telephone interviews with 100 graduates from each of the three program types (bachelors, diploma, and associates). Her method was to find, using local telephone directories and directory assistance, the telephone numbers for as many of the names on her lists as she could and to make calls until she had completed 100 interviews with graduates from each group. Thus, her final sample consisted of 300 recently graduated RNs.

Review and critique this research effort. Suggest alternative sampling designs. To assist you in your critique, use the questions below as well as the questions in Box 8-1 of the text.

a. What type of sampling design was used? Was this design appropriate? Would you recommend a different sampling approach? Why or why not? What are the advantages of the approach used? The disadvantages?

b. Identify what you believe to be the target and accessible populations in this study. How representative do you feel the accessible population is of the target population? How representative is the sample of this accessible population? What are some of the possible sources of sampling bias?

c. Did the research use a proportionate or disproportionate sampling plan? Is this appropriate? Why or why not?

d. Comment on the size of the sample. Does this sample size appear to be adequate?

3. Below are several suggested research articles. Read the introductory and methods sections of one or more of these articles and respond to parts **a** through **d** of Question D.2 in terms of these actual research studies.

- Adams, D., Miller, B. K., & Beck, L. (1996). Professionalism of hospital nurse executives and middle managers in 10 western states. *Western Journal of Nursing Research, 18,* 77–88.

- Berry, J. K., Vitalo, C. A., Larson, J. L., Patel, M., & Kim, M. J. (1996). Respiratory muscle strength in older adults. *Nursing Research, 45,* 154–159.

- Broom, B. L. (1994). Impact of marital quality and psychological well-being on parental sensitivity. *Nursing Research, 43,* 138–143.

- Simpson, T., Lee, E. R., & Cameron, C. (1996). Relationships among sleep dimensions and factors that impair sleep after cardiac surgery. *Research in Nursing & Health, 19,* 213–223.

4. A second brief summary of a fictitious study follows. Read the summary and then respond to the questions that follow.

Downie (1996) conducted an in-depth study of the emotional well-being of couples with fertility impairments. She conducted in-depth interviews with 10 couples who were undergoing infertility treatment in a private clinic, and compared them with 10 couples who had undergone such treatment and were expecting a baby. The interviews with the second group occurred in the fifth month of the pregnancies. In each of the two groups, the researcher began by selecting couples known to have had a range of experience with their fertility treatments (in terms of length and type of treatment and nature of the fertility impairment). Then, after the initial interviews were completed, the researcher recruited additional couples to saturate the theoretical lines that were developing within the data.

Review and critique this research effort. Suggest alternative sampling designs. To assist you in your critique, use the questions below as well as the questions in Box 8-2 of the text.

a. What type of sampling strategy was used?

b. Was this sampling strategy appropriate? Would you recommend a different sampling approach? Why or why not?

c. Comment on the size of the sample. Does this sample size appear to be adequate?

5. Below are several suggested research articles. Read the introductory and methods sections of one or more of these articles and respond to parts a through c of Question D.4 in terms of these actual research studies.

- Lear, D. (1996). "You're gonna be naked anyway": College students negotiating safer sex. *Qualitative Health Research, 6,* 112–134.

- MacEachen, E., & Munby, H. (1996). Developmentally disabled adults in community living: The significance of personal control. *Qualitative Health Research, 6,* 71–89.

- Roe, K. M., Minkler, M., & Barnwell, R. S. (1994). The assumption of caregiving: Grandmothers raising the children of the crack cocaine epidemic. *Qualitative Health Research, 4,* 281–303.

- Tarasuk, V., & Eakin, J. M. (1995). The problem of legitimacy in the experience of work-related back injury. *Qualitative Health Research, 5,* 204–221.

▨ E. SPECIAL PROJECTS

1. Suppose that you were interested in studying preventive health care behaviors among low-income urban residents. Describe how you might select a sample for your study using the following:

     a. A quota sample

     b. A cluster sample

     c. A typical case sample

     d. An extreme case sample

2. Propose a research question for a quantitative study. Specify a research and sampling design to study this problem. In particular, specify the following:

     a. The target population, including all criteria for inclusion in the population

     b. An accessible population

     c. A sampling design, together with a rationale

     d. A recommended sample size

With respect to b through d, be realistic. Take into account available resources, time, and level of expertise. That is, recommend a plan that would be feasible to implement.

Collection of Research Data

PART IV

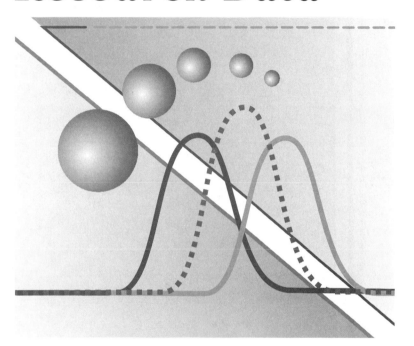

Chapter 9
Methods of Data Collection

◪ A. MATCHING EXERCISES

1. Match each descriptive statement from Set B with one of the statements from Set A. Indicate the letter corresponding to your response next to each item in Set B.

Set A

a. An interview
b. A questionnaire
c. Both an interview and a questionnaire
d. Neither an interview nor a questionnaire

Set B   *Responses*

1. Can provide respondents with the protection of anonymity   _____
2. Can be used with illiterate respondents   _____
3. Can contain both open- and closed-ended questions   _____
4. Is used in survey research   _____
5. Is the best way to measure human behavior   _____
6. Generally has high response rates   _____
7. Is generally an inexpensive method of data collection   _____
8. Is susceptible to response biases   _____

2. Match each problem statement from Set B with one of the statements from Set A. Indicate the letter corresponding to your response next to each item in Set B.

Set A

a. The study would *require* observational data
b. The study *could* use observational data, as well as other forms of data
c. The study is not amenable to observational data collection

Set B   *Responses*

1. Are nurses' attitudes toward abortion related to their years
    of nursing experience?   _____

2. Are patients' levels of stress related to their willingness to
    disclose their own fears to nursing staff?   _____

3. Are the crying patterns of infants related to their gestational
    age at birth?   _____

4. Is the degree of physical activity of a psychiatric patient related
    to his or her length of hospitalization?   _____

5. Are first-year nurses' ratings of effectiveness more highly related
    to their clinical grades or to their grades in academic courses
    while in nursing school?   _____

6. Is a child's fear during immunization related to the nurse's
    method of preparing the child for the shot?   _____

7. Does the presence of the father in the delivery room affect the
    mother's level of pain?   _____

8. Is the ability of dialysis patients to cleanse and dress their shunts
    related to their self-esteem?   _____

9. Is compliance with a medication regimen higher among women
    than men?   _____

10. Is aggressive behavior among hospitalized mentally retarded
    children related to styles of discipline by hospital staff?   _____

◩ B. COMPLETION EXERCISES

Write the words or phrases that correctly complete the sentences below.

1. One of the first decisions a researcher makes about research data is whether to
    collect new data or use _____.

2. _____ is the systematic gathering and criti-
    cal evaluation of data relating to past occurrences.

3. When data from a previous study are re-analyzed in a new study, this is re-
    ferred to as a _____.

4. The four dimensions along which data collection methods can vary are
    _____, _____,
    _____ , and _____
    _____.

5. In a focused interview, general question areas are normally prepared in the
    form of a _____.

6. When several respondents are assembled in one place to discuss questions, the
    approach being used is referred to as a _____.

7. A disadvantage of _____ questions is that the researcher may inadvertently omit some potentially important alternatives.

8. _____ questions are relatively inefficient in terms of the respondents' time.

9. A _____ is a trial run of a data-collection instrument to determine if it is soliciting the type and quality of information desired.

10. If respondents are not very verbal or articulate, _____ _____ questions are generally most appropriate.

11. A _____ is a device designed to assign scores to subjects to discriminate among them with respect to an attribute of interest.

12. Likert scales consist of a number of statements written in the _____ _____ form.

13. In Likert scales, positively worded statements are scored in one direction, and the scoring of negatively worded statements is _____ _____.

14. With a semantic differential, subjects are asked to rate concepts on a series of _____.

15. The bias introduced when respondents select options at either end of the response continuum is known as _____.

16. In Q sorts, forcing subjects to place a predetermined number of cards in each pile helps eliminate _____.

17. _____ are brief narrative descriptions of people or situations to which subjects are asked to react.

18. The major focus of observation in nursing research is on human _____ _____.

19. The problem of behavioral distortions arising when subjects are aware that they are being observed is known as _____.

20. The technique known as _____ involves the collection of unstructured observational data while the researcher participates in the activities of the group being observed.

21. The three major types of observational positioning in participant observation studies are _____, _____, and _____ positioning.

22. Data from unstructured observations are generally recorded on _____ and _____ _____.

23. In a structured observational setting, the most common procedure is to construct a(n) _____ for observed behaviors.

24. Biophysiologic measures that are taken directly within a living organism are _____ measures.

25. When physiologic materials are extracted from subjects and subjected to analysis, the data are referred to as _____ measures.

◩ C. STUDY QUESTIONS

1. Define the following terms. Use the textbook to compare your definition with the definition in Chapter 9 or in the Glossary.

a. Unstructured interview: _____

_____

b. Focused interview: _____

_____

c. Interview schedule: _____

_____

d. Questionnaire: _____

_____

e. Probing: _____

_____

f. Scale: _____

_____

g. Likert scale: _____

_____

h. Semantic differential: _____

_____

i. Visual analog scale: _____

_____

j. Response set biases: _____

_____

k. Social desirability response bias: _____

_____

l. Q sort: _____

_____

m. Projective technique: _____

n. Reactivity: _____

o. Participant observation: _____

p. Time sampling: _____

2. Below are several research problems. Indicate which type of unstructured self-report approach you might recommend using for each. Defend your response.

a. By what process do parents of a handicapped child learn to cope with their child's problem?

_____
_____

b. What are the barriers to preventive health care practices among the urban poor?

_____
_____

c. What stresses does the spouse of a terminally ill patient experience?

_____
_____

d. What types of information does a nurse draw on most heavily in formulating nursing diagnoses?

_____
_____

e. What are the health beliefs and health practices of elderly Native Americans living on a reservation?

_____
_____

3. Below are hypothetical responses of respondent Y and respondent Z to the Likert statements presented in Table 9-2 of the textbook. What would the total score for both of these respondents be, using the scoring rules described in Chapter 9?

Item No.	Respondent Y	Respondent Z
1	D	SA
2	A	D
3	SA	D
4	?	A
5	D	SA
6	SA	D
Total score:		

4. Below are hypothetical responses for respondents A, B, C, and D to the Likert statements presented in Table 9-2 of the text. Three of these four sets of responses contain some indication of a possible response set bias. Identify *which* three, and identify the types of bias.

Item No.	Respondent A	Respondent B	Respondent C	Respondent D
1	A	SA	SD	D
2	A	SD	SA	SD
3	SA	D	SA	D
4	A	A	SD	SD
5	SA	A	SD	SD
6	SA	SD	SA	D

5. Below are 10 attitudinal statements regarding attitudes toward natural family planning. For each statement, indicate how you think the item would be scored (*i.e.,* would "strongly agrees" be assigned a score of 1 or 5)? What are the maximum and minimum scores possible on this scale?

Statement	*Score for "Strongly Agree"*
a. Natural family planning is an effective method of avoiding unwanted pregnancies.	_____
b. Natural family planning removes the spontaneity from love making.	_____
c. Using natural family planning methods is too time-consuming.	_____

d. A man and a woman can be drawn   _____
   closer together by collaborating in
   using natural family planning.
e. Natural family planning is the safest   _____
   form of birth control.
f. Natural family planning is too risky if   _____
   one really doesn't want a pregnancy.
g. Natural family planning puts a woman   _____
   in better touch with her body.
h. Natural family planning is an accept-   _____
   able form of contraception.
i. All in all, natural family planning is the   _____
   best method of birth control developed.
j. Natural family planning is "unnatural"   _____
   in terms of the restrictions it imposes
   on a couple's intimacy.

6. Below are five statements that might appear on Q-sort cards. For each, describe different continua according to which the cards could be sorted (*e.g.,*
   one continuum could be "very much like me/not at all like me" for a statement
   such as "I like to go to parties").
a. Americans should be better educated   _____
   with respect to nutrition.
b. Nursing students need to understand   _____
   the fundamentals of research methods.
c. Insomnia   _____
d. Good fringe benefits   _____
e. A course on human sexual development   _____

7. Below are 10 research questions in which the dependent variable of interest is
   amenable to observation. Specify whether you think a structured or unstructured approach would be preferable and justify your response. Also, consider
   the extent to which reactivity might be a problem during the collection of observational data and make a recommendation regarding the degree to which
   the researcher should be concealed.
   a. What is the effect of touch on the crying behavior of hospitalized children?

   _____

   _____

   b. What is the effect of increased patient/staff ratios in psychiatric hospitals
      on interpersonal conflict among staff members?

   _____

   _____

c. Is the management of appetite loss in burn patients affected by nutritional information provided by nurses?

_____

_____

d. Is the amount and type of information transmitted at the change-of-shift report affected by the number of years of experience of the nurses?

_____

_____

e. Does a patient's need for personal space vary as a function of age?

_____

_____

f. Are the self-grooming activities of nursing home patients related to the frequency of visits from friends and relatives?

_____

_____

g. Is the adequacy of a student nurse's handwashing related to his or her type of educational preparation?

_____

_____

h. What is the process by which very low-birth-weight infants develop the sucking response?

_____

_____

i. What type of patient behaviors are most likely to elicit empathic behaviors in nurses?

_____

_____

j. Do nurses reinforce passive behaviors among female patients more than among male patients?

_____

_____

8. Indicate which of the measures below is an in vivo measure and which is an in vitro measure:

a. Blood pressure measures   _____

b. Electrocardiogram measures   _____

c. Hemoglobin concentration   _____

d. Total lung capacity   _____

e. Blood gas analysis of P_{CO_2} _____

f. Chronoscope measures   _____

g. Nasopharyngeal culture   _____

h. Goniometer readings   _____

i. Axillary temperature   _____

j. Blood pH   _____

9. Three nurse researchers were collaborating on a study of the effect of visits to surgical patients preoperatively by operating room nurses on the stress levels of those patients just before surgery. One researcher wanted to use the patients' self-reports on a standardized scale to measure stress; the second suggested using pulse rate; the third recommended the patients' white blood cell count. Which measure do you think would be the most appropriate for this research problem? Justify your response.

▧ D. APPLICATION EXERCISES

1. Below is a brief description of a fictitious study, followed by a critique. Do you agree with the critique? Can you add other comments relevant to issues discussed in Chapter 9 of the textbook? (Box 9-2 offers some guiding questions.)

> *Fictitious Study.* *O'Connell (1997) studied hospitalized patients' requests for nursing assistance in relation to their age, gender, and number of daily outside visitors. Her central hypothesis was that patient requests were higher among those with few or no visitors. Subjects for the study were 100 patients on a medical-surgical unit of a 500-bed hospital in New Hampshire. All 100 subjects were patients admitted for relatively routine procedures, such as appendectomies; none was terminally ill. Observations were made by the nursing staff, who were instructed to record verbatim all requests that the subjects made during a 24-hour period and all instances of patients' use of the call button. At the end of each shift, each nurse rated the patient on several dimensions, such as talkative/not talkative, hostile/friendly, and in no pain/in great pain.*
>
> *Each request was then categorized according to a sign system that O'Connell had developed. The categories included the following: request for medication; request for food or beverage; request for environmental change (e.g., temperature or light adjustment); request to see a physician; request for reading material, television, or radio; request for assistance (e.g., getting in/out of bed); and request for dialogue or emotional*

support. O'Connell performed all of the categorizations herself based on the nurses' verbatim accounts. O'Connell found that the number of patients' requests was unrelated to their gender and age, although there were age and gender differences in the types of request made. Patients with no visitors made significantly more requests than patients with one or more visitors on the day of the observation, and patients with no visitors were also somewhat more likely to be rated as unfriendly.

*   **Critique.** O'Connell's decision to use an observational approach seems appropriate. Self-reports (i.e., asking patients about the frequency and type of requests they had made) would have been subject to distortions arising from memory lapse and misreporting. Patients might also have a notion different from the researcher about what constitutes a request.*

*   O'Connell elected to use a highly structured observational scheme. This decision appears to have some merit: the investigator was interested in fairly specific phenomena that lent themselves to enumeration. It is also possible, however, that a more qualitative approach would have yielded additional insights regarding why patient requests were higher among those with no visitors.*

*   The use of both a category system and rating scales also seems to have been a good choice for capturing some information about the quantity and quality of patients' requests. The brief summary, however, does not provide a sufficient basis for evaluating whether the category system and dimensions for rating patients were appropriate. It would be useful to know how they were developed. Here again, a series of unstructured observations might have provided a rich basis for the development of relevant behavioral codes and dimensions of patient characteristics.*

*   Several other aspects of O'Connell's study could have been improved. First, consider the possibility of reactivity. It is likely that patients were not informed about their participation while the data were being collected, which in this case seems appropriate; the privacy of the patients was not seriously threatened, and patients would undoubtedly have altered their interactions with the nursing staff if they had known that their dialogue was being scrutinized. Thus, O'Connell's procedure of having nurses record patients' requests after they were made (i.e., after leaving the patients' rooms) eliminated the problem of reactivity stemming from the patient. But what about the reactivity of the nurses? The nurses knew exactly what the researcher was studying and could*

have communicated cues to the patients in subtle or not-so-subtle ways. The nurses' nonverbal behavior could have either encouraged or discouraged patients' requests for assistance.

Two other problems relate to the use of the nurses as the observational recorders. First, unless the nurses were thoroughly trained, some might have misinterpreted the researcher's definition of requests. Second, the nurses were required to report verbatim the patients' requests, an activity that is by no means easy, particularly for those whose main priority is patient care. In many cases, the nurses probably did not remember accurately the wording of the patients' questions.

From a methodologic point of view, the best procedure would have been to tape-record all nurse–patient dialogue unobtrusively. In addition to providing accuracy and eliminating the risk of nurse reactivity, the use of a recording device would have permitted more fine-grained analyses of the content and tone of the requests. However, concealed recording equipment would be ethically problematic. Perhaps the researcher could have told both the nursing staff and subjects about the presence of recording equipment and described only in broad terms the nature of the study (e.g., to understand patient–nurse communication patterns better).

O'Connell sampled an entire 24-hour period for all 100 subjects. It would probably have been wiser to sample 1-hour segments over a 48-hour to 72-hour interval. A single day may not have adequately represented the range of patient requests during a hospital stay and could also have been atypical in terms of visitation.

O'Connell elected to categorize patient communication that took the form of requests for assistance. The sign system covered all types of request, but no other patient conversation. Although the decision to use such a nonexhaustive category scheme is understandable, it does have the disadvantage of failing to provide a context for understanding patient behavior. If a patient made 15 requests in 1 day, it might be useful to know whether these requests represented all patient-initiated communication or only a small fraction of it.

Categorization of the requests according to a sign system was handled centrally by O'Connell rather than by individual nurse observers. This approach has the advantage of not having different biases produced by multiple observers. It does mean, however, that any biases went undetected. O'Connell would have been well-advised to have a second person catego-

rize the requests (or at least a portion of them) to determine agreement among different coders.

With respect to this latter issue, the use of nurses from all three shifts who rated patients' communication or to record actual dialogue would have provided yet another opportunity to verify nurses' observations independently. In summary, then, O'Connell's data collection plan was fairly well conceived but could also have been improved in a number of respects, including the judicious use of unstructured observations and possibly unstructured self-reports (e.g., interviews with patients who made many or few requests) to facilitate interpretation of the results.

2. Here is a brief summary of another fictitious study. Read the summary and then respond to the questions that follow.

Alongi (1996) conducted a survey that focused on drug use patterns in an urban adolescent population. The survey used self-administered questionnaires that were distributed to 25 high schools and administered in group (home room) sessions to 3568 respondents. The questionnaire consisted of 56 closed-ended and two open-ended questions. Included were background questions; questions on the students' attitudes toward, knowledge of, and experience with various drugs; and questions on the students' physical and mental health. The instrument was pretested with 10 college freshmen before administration.

Review and critique the above description of the overall study. Suggest possible alternative ways of collecting the data for this study. To assist you in your critique, here are some guiding questions. (Review also the critiquing guidelines in Box 9-1 of the textbook.)

a. The data in this study were collected by self-report. Could the data have been collected in another way? *Should* they have been, in your opinion?

b. Were the data collected by questionnaire or interview? Was the decision to use this method appropriate, or would you recommend an alternative procedure? Comment on the advantages and disadvantages of the procedure used for this particular research problem.

c. Comment on the degree of structure of the data collection approach. Would you recommend a more structured or a less structured approach? Why or why not?

d. Comment on the method in which the data were collected (*i.e.*, how was the instrument administered?). Was the method efficient? Did it yield an adequate response rate? Did it appear costly? What opportunity did respondents have to obtain clarifying information about the questions?

3. Below are several suggested research articles. Skim one of these articles, paying particular attention to the methods used to measure research variables and collect the data. Then respond to parts a to d of Question D.2 above in terms of this study.
   - Anderson, D. G. (1996). Homeless women's perceptions about their families of origin. *Western Journal of Nursing Research, 18,* 29–42.
   - Newens, A. J., McColl, E., Bond, S., & Priest, J. F. (1996). Patients' and nurses' knowledge of cardiac-related symptoms and cardiac misconceptions. *Heart & Lung, 25,* 190–199.
   - Porter, C. P., Oakley, D., Ronis, D. L., & Neal, R. W. (1996). Pathways of influence on fifth and eighth graders' reports about having had sexual intercourse. *Research in Nursing & Health, 19,* 193–204.
   - Shaw, C. R., Wilson, S. A., & O'Brien, M. E. (1994). Information needs prior to breast biopsy. *Clinical Nursing Research, 3,* 119–131.

4. Another brief summary of a fictitious study is presented next. Read the summary and then respond to the questions that follow.

   Lovely (1996) wanted to conduct a survey of nurses' attitudes toward abortion. For this study, she prepared 20 pro and con statements. After developing the items, she asked 10 of her colleagues to indicate their level of agreement or disagreement with the statements, on a seven-point scale. Lovely used the data from these 10 nurses as pretest data for refining the instrument. The original 20 items are presented below:

   1. *Every woman has a right to obtain an abortion if she does not want a baby.*
   2. *Abortion should be made available to women on demand.*
   *3. The government should subsidize the cost of abortions for poor women.
   4. *Abortions should be made illegal.*
   5. *The right to an abortion should be available to all women.*
   *6. Women whose lives are in danger because of their pregnancy should be allowed to have an abortion.
   7. *Abortion is morally wrong.*
   8. *Women need to have control of their own bodies by having abortion services available to them.*
   9. *Women who have abortions are murderers.*
   10. *People who oppose abortions have no compassion for women's circumstances.*
   11. *Legalizing abortion is a sign of the decay of civilization.*
   12. *No real woman would ever consider killing her own baby through abortion.*
   13. *The freedom to choose an abortion is essential to the liberation of women.*

14. *An enlightened society gives its citizens the right to make important choices, such as having an abortion.*

15. *The right to obtain a legal abortion should never be denied to women.*

16. *Women who have abortions deserve praise for their courage to make a tough decision.*

17. *No woman should be forced to bear a baby she does not want.*

*18. *If men had to bear babies, abortions would never have been illegal.*

19. *Abortion is one of the most despicable acts that a human can commit.*

20. *Having an abortion is better than having a child that would go unloved.*

On reviewing the pretest responses, Lovely eliminated items 3, 6, and 18 (indicated with an asterisk). She then had a 17-item scale ready to use in her survey.

Read and critique the description of Lovely's activities. Suggest possible alternative ways of collecting the data for the research problem. To assist you in your critique, some guiding questions are presented below.

a. What type of scale did the researcher develop?

b. Given the aims of the researcher, was the development of *any* type of scale appropriate? That is, could the data have been collected by another method? *Should* they have been, in your opinion?

c. Comment on the procedures used by the researcher to develop the scale. Was the scale adequately reviewed and pretested?

d. Critique the quality of the scale itself. Does it consist of a sufficient number of items? Is the number of response alternatives good? Does the scale do an adequate job of minimizing bias? If not, suggest modifications that might reduce response set biases.

e. Comment on why you think the items that were eliminated (items 3, 6, and 18) were removed from the final scale.

f. Do you think the researcher needed to develop this scale from scratch?

5. Another brief summary of a fictitious study is presented next. Read the summary and then respond to the questions that follow.

Bingham (1996) undertook an in-depth study of parents' experiences caring for children dying of cancer. The project was designed to describe the evolution of parents' caring practices in response to the demands of living with a dying child. Bingham conducted unstructured interviews with one or both parents separately, and then (in homes where there were two parents) another interview with the parents together. All interviews were tape-recorded and later transcribed for analysis. The researcher also spent 30 hours in each home in 10 separate sessions over a 2-month period observing parental caring practices. Most of the observations occurred in the child's bedroom or in a family/living room. The observations

focused on the following aspects of a caregiving episode: the
context for the episode; the nature and content of any interac-
tions; the activities that occurred; how the activities unfolded;
and what the outcomes of the activities were. All observational
notes were written out in full shortly after an observational
session, and the notes were later transcribed.

Review and critique this study. Suggest alternative ways of collecting the data
for the research problem. To assist you in your critique, here are some guiding
questions that focus primarily on the observational data. (Refer also to the
questions in Box 9-2 of the textbook.)

a. The data in this study were collected by observation (and interviews).
   Could the observational data have been collected in another way? *Should*
   they have been, in your opinion?

b. Would you classify the study as having used an unstructured or structured
   observational procedure? Was the amount of structure in the data collection appropriate, or should there have been more or less structure?

c. Specify the relationship between the observer and those being observed in
   terms of the degree to which the observer was concealed. Do you think that
   this relationship was appropriate? What kinds of problems might it create?

d. What types of observational bias do you think might be operational in this
   study?

6. Below are several suggested research articles in which an observational approach was used. Review one of the articles and respond to parts a to d of
Question D.5, to the extent possible, in terms of this study.

- Davis, T. M. A., Maguire, T. O., Haraphongse, M., & Schaumberger, M. R.
  (1994). Undergoing cardiac catheterization: The effects of informational
  preparation and coping style on patient anxiety during the procedure.
  Heart & Lung, 23, 140–150.

- Gross, D., Fogg, L., & Tucker, S. (1995). The efficacy of parent training for
  promoting positive parent-toddler relationships. *Research in Nursing &*
  Health, 18, 489–499.

- Miller, D. B. & Holditch-Davis, D. (1992). Interactions of parents and nurses
  with high-risk preterm infants. *Research in Nursing & Health, 15,* 187–197.

- Pickler, R. H., Frankel, H. B., Walsh, K. M., & Thompson, N. M. (1996). Effects of nonnutritive sucking on behavioral organization and feeding performance in preterm infants. *Nursing Research, 45,* 132–135.

7. Another brief summary of a fictitious study is presented next. Read the summary and then respond to the questions that follow.

Van Vlieberghe (1997) conducted a quasi-experimental study
of the effectiveness of a program for treating the physiologic
anemia associated with pregnancy. The experimental treat-
ment involved instruction regarding a nutritional regimen.
The experimental group received verbal instructions by a

nurse-midwife regarding dietary requirements and a list of foods known to be high in iron. Recommended daily amounts of certain foods were prescribed. The intervention also involved follow-up telephone conversations with the experimental group members at the 30th and 34th weeks of the pregnancy to discuss dietary and nutritional concerns. The comparison group members were given information that is normally given to pregnant women, with no individual follow-up. Fifty pregnant women who were outpatients at one hospital clinic served as the experimental subjects, and 50 pregnant women who were clients at an HMO served as the comparison group subjects. Van Vlieberghe chose hematocrit readings as the measure of effectiveness of the experimental intervention. During the 6th month of the pregnancy, and again at the 36th-week visit, a hematocrit laboratory test was performed. The data were analyzed by comparing the degree of change that had occurred in the two hematocrit readings within the two groups. The researcher found that there were no significant differences in physiologic anemia in the two groups, as measured by the changes in hematocrit tests.

Review and critique this study. Suggest alternative ways of collecting the data for the research problem. To assist you in your critique, here are some guiding questions. (Refer also to the questions in Box 9-3 of the textbook.)

a. The data in this study were collected by a biophysiologic measure. Could the data have been collected in another way? In your opinion, should they have been?

b. Is the measure used an in vivo or in vitro type of measurement? Is it an invasive or noninvasive type of procedure?

c. Comment on the objectivity of the data collection method. How does its objectivity compare with other methods of measuring the dependent variable (*e.g.,* observations of pallor of the skin, mucous membranes, and fingernail beds)?

d. What other biophysiologic measures might have been used to collect data in the study?

8. Below are several suggested research articles in which a biophysiologic measure was used. Review one of the articles and respond to parts a to d of Question D.7, to the extent possible, in terms of the study.

■ Bond, E. F., Heitkemper, M. M., & Jarrett, M. (1994). Intestinal transit and body weight responses to ovarian hormones and dietary fiber in rats. *Nursing Research, 43,* 18–24.

■ Green, L. A., & Froman, R. D. (1996). Blood pressure measurement during pregnancy: Auscultatory versus oscillatory methods. *Journal of Obstetric, Gynecologic, and Neonatal Nursing, 25,* 155–159.

- Wewers, M. E., Bowen, J. M., Stanlislaw, A. E., & Desimone, V. B. (1994). A nurse-delivered smoking cessation intervention among hospitalized postoperative patients. *Heart & Lung, 23,* 151–156.
- Zahr, L. K., & Balian, S. (1996). Responses of premature infants to routine nursing interventions and noise in the NICU. *Nursing Research, 44,* 179–185.

N E. SPECIAL PROJECTS

1. Develop a topic guide for studying barriers to health-care utilization among the urban poor.
2. Suggest one open-ended and one closed-ended question relating to each of the following variables. Compare the quality and amount of information that could be obtained with each.
   a. Women's attitudes toward nurse-midwives
   b. Factors influencing a decision to obtain a vasectomy
   c. Perceived adequacy of community health care services
   d. Student nurses' first experiences with the death of a patient
   e. Factors influencing nurses' administration of pain-relieving narcotics to patients
3. Suppose that you were interested in studying hospitalized patients' satisfaction with their nursing care. Develop five positively worded and five negatively worded statements that could be used to construct a Likert scale for such a study.
4. Below is a list of five variables. Indicate briefly how you might operationalize each using structured observational procedures.
   a. Fear in hospitalized children
   b. Pain during childbirth
   c. Dependency in psychiatric patients
   d. Empathy in nursing students
   e. Cooperativeness in chemotherapy patients
5. Develop a research question for a study that could use observational data collection procedures. Make a recommendation regarding the use of a structured or unstructured approach for this problem.
6. Suppose that you wanted to evaluate the effect of an experimental nursing intervention on the well-being and comfort of cardiac patients. Indicate several physiologic measures you might consider using in such a study. Evaluate each of your suggestions with respect to ease of obtaining the data, relevance, and objectivity.
7. Using procedures described in Chapter 9, suggest methods of collecting data on the following: fear of death among the elderly; body image among amputees; reactions to the onset of menarche; nurses' morale in an emergency room; and dependence among cerebral-palsied children.

Chapter 10
Data Quality Assessments

◤ A. MATCHING EXERCISES

1. Match each statement from Set B with one of the phrases from Set A. Indicate the letter corresponding to your response next to each of the statements in Set B.

Set A

a. Reliability
b. Validity
c. Both reliability and validity
d. Neither reliability nor validity

Set B   *Responses*

1. Is concerned with the accuracy of quantitative measures   _____
2. The measures must be high on this for the results of a
   quantitative study to be valid   _____
3. If a quantitative measure possesses this, it is necessarily valid _____
4. Can in some cases be estimated by procedures that yield a
   quantified coefficient   _____
5. Can be enhanced by lengthening (adding subparts to) a scale   _____
6. Is necessarily high when the measure is high on objectivity   _____
7. Is concerned with whether the researcher has adequately
   conceptualized the variables under investigation   _____
8. Equivalence is one aspect of this   _____

2. Match each statement from Set B with one of the phrases from Set A. Indicate the letter corresponding to your response next to each of the statements in Set B.

Set A

a. Data triangulation
b. Investigator triangulation
c. Theory triangulation
d. Method triangulation

Set B   ***Responses***

1. A researcher studying health beliefs of the rural elderly interviews old people and health care providers in the area.   _____

2. A researcher tests narrative data, collected in interviews with people who attempted suicide, against two alternative explanations of stress and coping.   _____

3. Two researchers independently interview 10 informants in a study of adjustment to a cancer diagnosis, and debrief with each other to review what they have learned.   _____

4. A researcher studying school-based clinics observes interactions in the clinics and also conducts in-depth interviews with students.   _____

5. A researcher studying the process of resolving an infertility problem interviews husbands and wives separately.   _____

6. Themes emerging in the field notes of an observer on a psychiatric ward are categorized and labeled independently by the researcher and an assistant.   _____

▧ B. COMPLETION EXERCISES

Write the words or phrases that correctly complete the sentences below.

1. People are not measured directly; their _____ are measured.

2. The procedure known as _____ refers to the assignment of numeric information to indicate how much of an attribute is present.

3. In measurement, numbers are assigned according to specified _____ _____.

4. Obtained scores almost always consist of an error component and a _____ _____ component.

5. From a measurement perspective, response set biases represent a source of _____.

6. A reliable measure is one that maximizes the _____ _____ component of observed scores.

7. Test–retest reliability focuses on the _____ of a measure.

8. The internal consistency of a measure can be assessed through a procedure known as the _____ technique, which involves dividing the items of an instrument into two parts.

9. Another term for internal consistency is _____.

10. Procedures that examine the proportion of agreements between two independent judges yield estimates of _____.

11. An instrument that is not reliable cannot be _____.

12. A measure that looks as though it is measuring what it purports to measure is said to have _____ validity.

13. The type of validity that focuses on the representativeness of the subparts of a measure is _____ validity.

14. The type of validity that deals with the ability of an instrument to distinguish people who differ in terms of some future criterion is _____ _____ validity.

15. The four criteria for establishing the trustworthiness of qualitative data are _____, _____, _____, and _____ _____.

16. When a qualitative researcher undertakes a _____ _____ in the field, he or she has more opportunity to develop trust with informants and to test for possible misinformation.

17. The use of multiple sources of information in a study as a means of verification is known as _____.

18. The technique of debriefing with informants to evaluate the credibility of qualitative data is referred to as _____.

19. The criterion of _____ refers to the objectivity or neutrality of the data.

20. In qualitative studies, a(n) _____ of data and documents by an independent reviewer can verify the dependability and neutrality of the data and their interpretation.

▨ C. STUDY QUESTIONS

1. Define the following terms. Use the textbook to compare your definition with the definition in Chapter 10 or in the Glossary.

   a. Measurement: _____
   _____

   b. Obtained score: _____
   _____

   c. Error of measurement: _____
   _____

d. Reliability: _____

_____

e. Test–retest reliability: _____

_____

f. Reliability coefficient: _____

_____

g. Internal consistency: _____

_____

h. Split-half technique: _____

_____

i. Cronbach's alpha: _____

_____

j. Interrater reliability: _____

_____

k. Validity: _____

_____

l. Content validity: _____

_____

m. Criterion-related validity: _____

_____

n. Construct validity: _____

_____

o. Known-groups technique: _____

_____

p. Triangulation: _____

_____

q. Transferability of data: _____

_____

r. Audit trail: _____

_____

s. Psychometric evaluation: _____

_____

2. The reliability of measures of which of the following attributes would not be appropriately assessed using a test–retest procedure with 1 week between administrations? Why?

a. Attitudes toward abortion:

_____

_____

  b. Stress:

_____

_____

  c. Achievement motivation:

_____

_____

  d. Nursing effectiveness:

_____

_____

  e. Depression:

_____

_____

3. Comment on the meaning and implications of the following statement.

A researcher found that the internal consistency of her 20-item scale measuring attitudes toward nurse-midwives was .74, using the Cronbach alpha formula.

4. In the situation described below, what might some of the sources of measurement error be?

A sample of 100 nurses who worked in a large metropolitan hospital were asked to complete a 10-item Likert scale designed to measure job satisfaction. The questionnaires were distributed by nursing supervisors at the end of shifts. The staff nurses were asked to complete the forms and return them immediately to their supervisors.

5. Identify what is incorrect about the following statements:

  a. "My scale is highly reliable, so it must be valid."

_____

_____

  b. "My instrument yielded an internal consistency coefficient of .80, so it must be stable."

_____

_____

  c. "The validity coefficient between my scale and a criterion measure was .40; therefore, my scale must be of low validity."

_____

_____

d. "The validation study proved that my measure has construct validity."

_____

_____

e. "My advisor examined my new measure of dependence in nursing home residents and, based on its content, assured me the measure was valid."

_____

_____

◩ D. APPLICATION EXERCISES

1. Below is a brief description of a fictitious study, followed by a critique. Do you agree with the critique? Can you add other comments relevant to issues discussed in Chapter 10 of the textbook? (Box 10-1 offers some guiding questions.)

Fictitious Study. *Fox (1996) developed a scale that measured feelings of loneliness and social isolation among the elderly. She developed 12 Likert statements, six of which were worded positively and the other six of which were worded negatively. Examples include, "I have lots of friends with whom I am close" and "Sometimes days go by without my having a real conversation with someone." Fox pretested her instrument with 50 men and women aged 60 to 70 years living independently in the community. She estimated the reliability of the scale using internal consistency procedures (Cronbach's alpha), which yielded a reliability coefficient of .61.*

Fox took two steps to validate her scale. First, she asked two geriatric nurses to examine the 12 items to assess the scale's content validity. These experts suggested some wording changes on three items and recommended replacing one other. Next, she compared the scale scores of 100 elderly widows and widowers with those of 100 elderly married men and women. Her rationale was that the widowed would probably feel lonelier as a group than the nonwidowed. Her expectation was confirmed. Fox concluded that her scale was reasonably valid and reliable.

__Critique.__ Fox took some reasonable steps in constructing her scale and assessing its quality. For example, Fox's scale was counterbalanced for negative and positive statements, thereby reducing the risk of measurement error attributable to such response sets as the acquiescence response bias. It appears that she included a sufficient number of items (12) to

*yield discriminating scores. She used the Cronbach's alpha
approach, which is the best method available for assessing the
internal consistency of Likert scales.*

*The reliability of Fox's scale, however, could and should
be improved. The reliability coefficient of .61 suggests that
there is considerable measurement error. There are several
steps that Fox could take to try to raise the reliability. First,
she could make sure that each item on her scale is doing the
job it was intended to do. Remember that scales are designed
to discriminate among people who possess different amounts
of some trait, in this case social isolation. If Fox identifies one
or more items for which there is little variability (i.e., most respondents either agree or disagree), then the item should be
discarded. It is probably not measuring social isolation if
everyone responds the same way.*

*Next, Fox could make sure that her scoring procedure is
correct. Her assignment of scores is based on a judgment of
what is a positively and negatively worded item. Respondents
with high scores should agree with the positively worded
items and disagree with the negatively worded ones. If substantial numbers of people did the opposite, either the item
should be eliminated or perhaps the scoring should be reversed. If people with high scores are divided in their agreement with an item, this could be caused by ambiguity in the
wording of that question, so perhaps it should be revised. Finally, Fox should consider lengthening the scale. Other things
being equal, longer scales are more reliable than shorter ones.*

*Fox's efforts to validate her scale also deserve comment.
Her first step was to consider the content validity of the scale.
Having two knowledgeable people examine the scale was a
very desirable thing to do. Nevertheless, it cannot be said that
this activity in itself ensured the validity of the scale. Content
validity is not as relevant for social–psychological scales as it
is for, say, achievement tests. For variables such as social isolation, there is simply no well-defined domain from which
items can be sampled. If Fox had used only the content validity approach, she would have done little to establish her scale's
validity.*

*As a second step, Fox used the known-groups technique.
The data she obtained provided some useful evidence of the
scale's construct validity. After making some of the revisions
suggested above to improve the scale's reliability, however,
Fox would do well to gather some additional data to support*

the scale's validity. For example, one might suspect that people would feel less socially isolated if they reported having kin living within a 20-mile radius; if they had visited with a friend within a 72-hour period preceding the completion of the scale; and if they were active members of a club, church group, or other social organization. If Fox took these additional steps to establish the reliability and validity of her scale and obtained favorable results, she could be justifiably confident that the quality of her scale was high.

2. Here is a brief summary of another fictitious study. Read the summary and then respond to the questions that follow.

Gardner (1996) wanted to study paternal bonding and attachment among men who had recently become fathers. Her main objective was to compare paternal attachment among men who had participated with their wives in prenatal classes and were present during childbirth with men who had not. In reviewing prior work in this area, Gardner was unable to identify a paternal attachment scale that she found suitable to her needs. Therefore, she developed her own scale to measure paternal attachment. Her scale consisted of 10 statements that respondents were asked to rate as "very much like me," "somewhat like me," or "not at all like me." An example of the statements on the scale is: "The birth of my baby aroused sentiments of immediate affection, closeness, and pride." Total scores were obtained by using procedures analogous to those used for summated rating scales.

Gardner pretested her scale with 30 men within 48 hours of the delivery of their babies. The internal consistency of the scale was assessed using the split-half technique, which yielded a reliability coefficient of .68. In terms of validating the instrument, Gardner used two approaches. First, she invited two colleagues who worked in maternal-child nursing to review the 10 statements and evaluate them in terms of content validity. Second, she asked nurses who worked in the hospital maternity ward to provide ratings, on a 0-to-10 scale, of how attached each new father appeared to be, based on the nurses' observations of the fathers' behavior with regard to their babies. The correlation between the fathers' scale scores and the nurses' ratings was .56.

Review and critique this research effort. Suggest alternative ways of assessing the quality of the data collection instrument. To assist you in your critique, answer the guiding questions below. (Refer also to the relevant critiquing guidelines in Box 10-1 of the textbook.)

a. What method was used to assess the reliability of the instrument? On what aspect of reliability does this method focus? Is this focus appropriate? Should some alternative method for estimating reliability have been used? Should an *additional* method of estimating reliability have been used?

b. Comment on the adequacy of the instrument's reliability. Should the reliability be better? If so, what might the researcher do to improve the reliability?

c. What method was used to assess the validity of the instrument? On what aspect of validity does this approach focus? Is this focus appropriate? Should some alternative method for estimating validity have been used? Should an *additional* method of estimating validity have been used?

d. Comment on the adequacy of the instrument's validity. Should the validity be better? If so, what might the researcher do to improve the validity?

3. Below are several suggested research articles. Read one of these articles, paying special attention to the ways the researcher assessed the adequacy of his or her measuring tool. Evaluate the measurement strategy, using parts a to d of Question D.1 as a guide. (Ignore the more technical aspects of the report, such as those that deal with factor analysis.)

- Carruth, A. K. (1996). Development and testing of the caregiver reciprocity scale. *Nursing Research, 45,* 92–97.

- Hill, P. D., & Humenick, S. S. (1996). Development of the H & H Lactation Scale. *Nursing Research, 45,* 136–140.

- Lareau, S. C., Carrieri-Kohlman, V., Janson-Bjerklie, S., & Roos, P. J. (1994). Development and testing of the Pulmonary Functional Status and Dyspnea Questionnaire (PFSDQ). *Heart & Lung, 23,* 242–250.

- Martin, L. L. (1994). Validity and reliability of a quality-of-life instrument: The Chronic Respiratory Disease Questionnaire. *Clinical Nursing Research, 3,* 146–156.

- Norwood, S. L. (1996). The Social Support Apgar: Instrument development and testing. *Research in Nursing & Health, 19,* 143–152.

4. Below are several suggested research reports on qualitative studies. Read one of the articles, paying special attention to the ways in which the researcher addressed data quality issues. Use the relevant guidelines in Box 10-2 to assist you in your appraisal of the data's trustworthiness and the researcher's efforts to document it.

- Beck, C. T. (1992). The lived experience of postpartum depression: A phenomenological study. *Nursing Research, 41,* 166–170.

- Bright, M. A. (1992). Making place: The first birth in an intergenerational family context. *Qualitative Health Research, 2,* 75–98.

- Collins, B. A., McCoy, S. A., Sale, S., & Weber, S. E. (1994). Descriptions of comfort by substance-using and nonusing postpartum women. *Journal of Obstetric, Gynecologic, and Neonatal Nursing, 23,* 293–302.

- Stuhlmiller, C. M. (1994). Occupational meanings and coping practices of rescue workers in an earthquake disaster. *Western Journal of Nursing Research, 16,* 301–316.

◪ E. SPECIAL PROJECTS

1. Develop a problem statement (or a hypothesis) for a nursing research study that would require a quantitative data collection approach. Prepare operational definitions that specify measurement rules for the variables in your statement.

2. Suppose that you were developing an instrument to measure attitudes toward test-tube babies. Your measure consists of 15 Likert-type items. Describe what you would do to (a) estimate the reliability of your scale and (b) assess the validity of your scale.

3. Suggest the type of groups that might be used to validate measures of the following concepts using the known-groups technique:

a. Self-esteem
b. Empathy
c. Capacity for self-care
d. Emotional dependence
e. Depression

4. Suppose you were interested in conducting an in-depth study of women who had been raped. Describe ways in which you might achieve (a) data triangulation, (b) method triangulation, (c) member checks.

Analysis of
Research Data

PART V

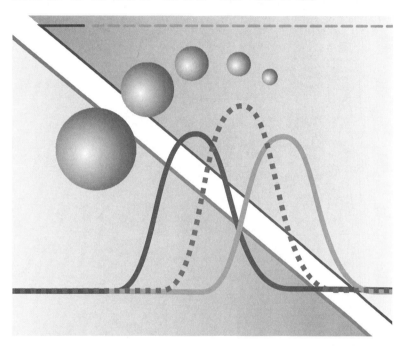

Chapter 11
Quantitative Analysis

◩ A. MATCHING EXERCISES

1. Match each variable in Set B with the level of measurement from Set A that captures the highest possible level for that variable. Indicate the letter corresponding to your response next to each variable in Set B.

Set A

a. Nominal scale
b. Ordinal scale
c. Interval scale
d. Ratio scale

Set B   *Responses*

1. Hours spent in labor before childbirth   _____
2. Religious affiliation   _____
3. Time to first postoperative voiding   _____
4. Responses to a single Likert scale item   _____
5. Temperature on the centigrade scale   _____
6. Nursing specialty area   _____
7. Status on the following scale: in poor health; in fair health; in
   good health; in excellent health   _____
8. Pulse rate   _____
9. Score on a 25-item Likert scale   _____
10. Highest college degree attained (bachelor's, master's, doctorate)   _____
11. Apgar scores   _____
12. Membership in the American Nurses' Association   _____

2. Match each statement or phrase from Set B with one of the phrases from Set A. Indicate the letter corresponding to your response next to each of the statements in Set B.

Set A

a. Measure(s) of central tendency
b. Measure(s) of variability
c. Measure(s) of neither central tendency nor variability
d. Measure(s) of both central tendency and variability

Set B   *Responses*

1. The range   _____
2. In lay terms, an average   _____
3. A percentage   _____
4. A parametric statistic   _____
5. Descriptor(s) of a distribution of scores   _____
6. Descriptor(s) of how heterogeneous a set of values is   _____
7. The standard deviation   _____
8. The mode   _____
9. Is normally positively skewed   _____
10. The median   _____

3. Match each phrase or statement from Set B with one of the phrases in Set A. Indicate the letter corresponding to your response next to each of the statements in Set B.

Set A

a. Parametric test
b. Nonparametric test
c. Neither parametric nor nonparametric tests
d. Both parametric and nonparametric tests

Set B   *Responses*

1. The chi-squared test   _____
2. Paired *t*-test   _____
3. Researcher establishes the risk of Type I errors   _____
4. Used when a score distribution is nonnormal   _____
5. Offers proof that the null hypothesis is either true or false _____
6. Assumes the dependent variable is measured on an interval or ratio scale   _____
7. Uses sample data to estimate population values   _____
8. ANOVA *F*-ratio   _____
9. Computed statistics are compared with tabled values based on theoretical distributions   _____
10. Used when there is only one variable   _____

4. Match each phrase from Set B with one (or more) of the statistical analyses presented in Set A. Indicate the letter corresponding to your response next to each of the statements in Set B.

Set A

a. Multiple regression analysis
b. Discriminant function analysis
c. Factor analysis
d. Logistic regression
e. Multivariate analysis of variance

Set B   *Responses*

1. Has more than one independent variable   _____
2. Yields an R^2 statistic   _____
3. Used to reduce variables to a smaller number of dimensions   _____
4. Has more than one dependent variable   _____
5. Is a multivariate statistical procedure   _____
6. Involves a dependent variable that is categorical (nominal level) _____
7. Translates the probability of an event occurring into an odds ratio _____
8. Is sometimes called MANOVA   _____

▨ B. COMPLETION EXERCISES

Write the words or phrases that correctly complete the sentence below.

1. Nominal measurement involves a simple _____ of objects according to some criterion.

2. Rank-order questions are an example of _____ measures.

3. With ratio-level measures, there is a real, rational _____ _____.

4. Unlike ordinal measures, interval measures involve _____ _____ between points on the scale.

5. A descriptive index (*e.g.,* percentage) from a population is called a(n) _____ _____.

6. A(n) _____ is a systematic arrangement of quantitative data from lowest to highest values.

7. _____ are a common way of presenting frequency information in graphic form.

8. A distribution is described as _____ if the two halves are *mirror* images of each other.

9. A distribution is described as _____ skewed if its longer tail points to the left.

10. A distribution that has only one peak is said to be _____
_____.

11. Many human characteristics, such as height and intelligence, are distributed to approximate a(n) _____.

12. Measures that summarize the typical value in a distribution are known as measures of _____.

13. Measures of _____ are concerned with how spread out the data are.

14. When scores are not very spread out (*i.e.,* dispersed over a wide range of values), the sample is said to be _____ with respect to that variable.

15. The most widely used measure of variability is the _____
_____.

16. Descriptive statistics for two variables examined simultaneously are called _____
_____.

17. Relationships are described as _____ if high values on one variable are associated with low values on a second.

18. The most commonly used correlation index is _____
_____.

19. Researchers using quantitative analysis apply _____
_____ to draw conclusions about a population based on information from a sample.

20. Sampling distributions of means have a _____ distribution.

21. The degree of risk of making a _____ error is controlled by the researcher.

22. Tests that involve the estimation of parameters are referred to as _____ tests.

23. The most commonly used _____ are the .05 and .01 levels.

24. Using $\alpha = .01$ rather than $\alpha = .05$ level *increases* the risk of committing a _____ error.

25. The statistic computed in an analysis of variance is the _____
_____ statistic.

26. When both the independent and dependent variables are nominal measures, the test statistic usually calculated is the _____.

27. The square of _____ indicates the proportion of variance accounted for in a dependent variable by several independent variables.

28. ANCOVA is shorthand for _____.

29. In ANCOVA, the extraneous variable being controlled is referred to as the _____.

30. In factor analysis, the underlying dimensions of a large set of variables are referred to as _____.

31. The first phase in factor analysis is the _____ in which the original variables are condensed into a smaller number of factors.

32. MANOVA is the acronym for _____.

▧ C. STUDY QUESTIONS

1. Define the following terms. Use the textbook to compare your definition with the definition in Chapter 11 or in the Glossary.

   a. Level of measurement: _____
   _____

   b. Statistic: _____
   _____

   c. Skewed distribution: _____
   _____

   d. Bimodal distribution: _____
   _____

   e. Normal distribution: _____
   _____

   f. Median: _____
   _____

   g. Mean: _____
   _____

   h. Standard deviation: _____
   _____

   i. Correlation coefficient: _____
   _____

   j. Sampling error: _____
   _____

   k. Sampling distribution: _____
   _____

l. Standard error of the mean: _____

m. Type I error: _____

n. Type II error: _____

o. Level of significance: _____

p. Statistical significance: _____

q. Nonparametric tests: _____

r. *t*-test: _____

s. Analysis of variance: _____

t. Chi-squared test: _____

u. Multivariate statistics: _____

v. Multiple regression analysis: _____

w. Analysis of covariance: _____

x. Factor analysis: _____

y. Discriminant function analysis: _____

z. Logistic regression: _____

2. Name five physiologic measures that yield ratio-level measurements.

a. _____

b. _____

c. _____

d. _____

e. _____

3. Prepare a frequency distribution and frequency polygon for the set of scores below, which represent the ages of 30 women receiving estrogen replacement therapy:

47 50 51 50 48 51 50 51 49 51
54 49 49 53 51 52 51 52 50 53
49 51 52 51 50 55 48 54 53 52

Describe the resulting distribution in terms of its symmetry and modality (*i.e.,* whether it is unimodal or multimodal).

4. Calculate the mean, median, and mode for the following pulse rates:

78 84 69 98 102 72 87 75 79 84 88 84 83 71 73

Mean: _____
Median: _____
Mode: _____

5. A group of nurse researchers measured the amount of time (in minutes) spent in recreational activities by a sample of 200 hospitalized paraplegic patients. They compared male and female patients as well as those aged 50 and younger versus those older than over 50 years. The four group means (50 subjects per group) were as follows:

Age	Male	Female
≤50 years	98.2	70.1
>50 years	50.8	68.3

A two-way ANOVA yielded the following results:

	F	*df*	*p*
Sex	3.61	1,196	NS
Age group	5.87	1,196	<.05
Sex × Age group	6.96	1,196	<.01

Interpret the meaning of these results.

6. The correlation between the number of days absent per year and annual salary in a sample of 100 employees of an insurance company was found to be $-.23$ ($p < .05$). Discuss this result in terms of its meaning.

7. Indicate which statistical tests you would use to analyze data for the following variables:

a. Variable 1 is psychiatric patients' gender; variable 2 is whether the patient has attempted suicide in the past 6 months.

b. Variable 1 is the participation versus nonparticipation of patients with a pulmonary embolus in a special treatment group; variable 2 is the pH of the patients' arterial blood gases.

c. Variable 1 is serum creatinine concentration levels; variable 2 is daily urine output.

d. Variable 1 is patients' marital status (married versus divorced/separated/widowed versus never married); variable 2 is the patients' degree of self-reported depression (measured on a 30-item depression scale).

8. Suggest possible covariates that could be used to control extraneous variation in the following analyses:

a. An analysis of the effect of family income on the incidence of child abuse:

b. An analysis of the effect of age on patients' acceptance of pastoral counseling:

c. An analysis of the effect of therapeutic touch on patients' anxiety levels:

d. An analysis of the effect of need for achievement on students' attrition from a nursing program:

_____

_____

e. An analysis of the effect of faculty rank on faculty members' satisfaction with communications among colleagues:

_____

_____

9. In the following examples, which multivariate procedure is most appropriate for analyzing the data?

a. A researcher is testing the effect of verbal expressiveness, self-esteem, age, and the availability of family supports among a group of recently discharged psychiatric patients on recidivism (_i.e.,_ whether they will be readmitted within 12 months after discharge).

_____

_____

b. A researcher is comparing the bereavement and coping processes of recently widowed and divorced individuals, controlling for their age.

_____

_____

c. A researcher wants to test the effects of two drug treatments and two dosages of each drug on blood pressure, and the pH and Po_2 levels of arterial blood gases.

_____

_____

d. A researcher wants to predict hospital staff absentee rates based on month of the year, staff rank, shift, number of years with the hospital, and marital status.

_____

_____

10. Below is a list of variables that a nurse researcher might be interested in predicting. For each, suggest at least three independent variables that could be used in a multiple regression analysis.

a. Leadership in nursing supervisors: _____

_____

b. Nurses' frequency of administering pain medication: _____

    c. Proficiency in doing patient interviews: _____

_____

    d. Patient satisfaction with nursing care: _____

_____

    e. Anxiety levels of prostatectomy patients: _____

_____

◩ D. APPLICATION EXERCISES

1. Below is a brief description of a fictitious study, followed by a critique. Do you agree with the critique? Can you add other comments relevant to issues discussed in Chapter 11 of the textbook? (Box 11-1 offers some guiding questions.)

> ***Fictitious Study.*** *Carroll (1996) studied psychological distress and marital satisfaction in a sample of infertile and sterile couples. He hypothesized that levels of well-being and satisfaction would be related to whether the source of the fertility problem was the person himself or herself or the person's partner. He also hypothesized that, overall, women would be more adversely affected than men by the fertility problem. Carroll's sample consisted of 100 couples who were patients at an infertility clinic—50 couples for whom infertility had been diagnosed as attributable to male factors and 50 for whom infertility was attributable to female factors.*
>
>   *Table 11-A is Carroll's table summarizing the demographic characteristics of the four groups of subjects. Carroll administered a questionnaire to all 200 subjects. The questionnaire included 45 Likert-type questions, which Carroll used to create three psychological scales, labeled as follows: (1) depression, (2) marital satisfaction, and (3) feelings of gender-role inadequacy. The scores on the three scales were analyzed in three separate two-way (2 × 2) ANOVAs, with gender and source of the fertility problem as the independent variables. Table 11-B summarizes the results of Carroll's analyses. Carroll concluded on the basis of these data that his hypotheses were partially supported.*
>
>   ***Critique.*** *Carroll used Table 11-A to present some basic background information about the four groups of subjects in his study. The table specifies for each group the mean and standard deviation for four variables that were not used in testing the research hypotheses but that provide the reader with a picture of the subjects. The mean and standard deviation appear to be the appropriate indexes for most of the char-*

Table 11-A. Major Characteristics of the Research Sample

	Personal Infertility				Partner Infertility			
	Males		Females		Males		Females	
Characteristic	X	SD	X	SD	X	SD	X	SD
Age	28.7	3.2	29.8	5.4	30.2	4.6	25.4	2.8
Number of years of education	13.2	1.7	11.8	1.3	13.6	2.0	12.0	1.5
Number of children	.2	.1	.1	.1	.7	.3	.4	.2
Number of years married	5.2	1.3	4.2	.9	4.2	.9	5.2	1.3
Number of subjects	50		50		50		50	

*acteristics, although the use of percentages would probably
have been more illuminating in the case of the variable number of children. For example, it would have been more useful
to know that 10% of the men with a fertility problem had previously fathered a child. The mean value of .2 children could
be distorted because some of the men may have fathered several children, and most may have never been a parent. The
columns and rows in Table 11-A are clearly labeled so that we*

Table 11-B. Summary of Analysis of Variance Results

Dependent Variable	Source of Fertility Problem	Mean Scores		F-Test Results
		Males	Females	
Depression scale scores	Self	20.1	29.1	Sex: $F = 5.9, p < .05$
	Partner	15.3	23.6	Source: $F = 6.7, p < .01$
				Sex × Source: $F = 1.9$, NS
Marital satisfaction scale scores	Self	25.6	26.3	Sex: $F = 1.1$, NS
	Partner	28.7	24.9	Source: $F = 0.9$, NS
				Sex × Source: $F = 1.3$, NS
Sex role inadequacy scale scores	Self	27.5	38.9	Sex: $F = 6.4, p < .05$
	Partner	19.5	22.8	Source: $F = 9.3, p < .01$
				Sex × Source: $F = 4.9, p < .05$

can look up a piece of information fairly easily. For example, the mean age of women who had a fertility problem was 29.8, whereas the mean age of women whose partners had a fertility problem was 25.4. Although the layout of the table is acceptable as presented, the reader might have found it easier to interpret the information if the groups had been reordered so that the male and female partners in a couple were in adjacent columns. In the current version, the men in the first column are married to the women in the fourth column, so that the format makes it difficult to understand couple characteristics.

Carroll used inferential statistics to test his research hypotheses and succinctly summarized a considerable amount of information about the results in Table 11-B. The table tells us the mean scale scores for the three dependent variables for all four groups of subjects. Standard deviations were not presented, but it is possible that there were few group differences in variability and that the overall standard deviations were therefore reported in the text of the research report. The table also tells us the value of the F statistic and the level of significance of the test for both the main and interaction effects. Degrees of freedom are not specified, presumably because they were the same for all tests.

Carroll's choice of a two-way ANOVA seems fairly well suited to his research design, hypotheses, and measures. His design called for the collection of data from both partners of 100 couples, half of whom were diagnosed as having a male-based fertility problem, and the other half a female-based problem. His hypotheses involved both the gender-of-subject factor and a source-of-problem factor. His measures involved two nominal-level independent variables (gender and source of problem) and interval-level dependent variables (the scale scores). The use of a parametric procedure seems justified, although if we had more information about the distribution of the scale scores we might learn that the distributions were too skewed to justify parametric statistical tests.

Carroll did not use any multivariate statistics, but he might well have done so. For example, there is no indication that factor analysis was used to analyze the underlying dimensionality of the 45 Likert items. The scales were apparently created based on the researcher's judgment. Such judgments are frequently erroneous, however. A factor analysis might have shown that there were really four (or more) important dimensions being tapped by the 45 Likert statements. The use of four rather than three dependent variables could alter the nature of the researcher's findings and conclusions.

Other multivariate procedures might also have been appropriate. For example, ANCOVA could have been used to control such extraneous variables as age, socioeconomic status, and parenting history of the subjects. Table 11-A suggests, for example, that there was some variability among the four groups in terms of these characteristics. Controlling them could alter the findings and lead to different conclusions about the relationship between the independent variables and the dependent variables.

The results of Carroll's study indicated that the women were significantly more depressed and felt less adequate about their gender roles than their husbands (regardless of the source of the fertility problem), consistent with his hypothesis. Also as hypothesized, the person who was the source of the fertility problem was more depressed and had greater feelings of gender-role inadequacy than the person's partner (regardless of gender). Differences relating to marital satisfaction were not statistically significant; the observed differences on this scale were probably the result of random fluctuations only. Thus, Carroll's hypothesis regarding marital satisfaction was not supported by the data.

Although not specifically hypothesized, there was one more significant effect: on the gender-role inadequacy scale, the interaction between gender and source of the problem was significant at the .05 level. An inspection of the means shows that this interaction does not involve a crossover effect. In the example shown in Table 11-12 of the textbook, it may be recalled, an interaction was observed: freshmen students had higher test scores when exposed to the lecture, whereas sophomore students had higher test scores when exposed to the film. In Carroll's data, the interaction is somewhat different. We can interpret the results as follows: overall, the women had more negative gender-role feelings than the men; overall, the people who were the source of the fertility problem felt worse about gender-role inadequacy than those whose partners were the source; but being a woman and being the source of the fertility problem had a compounding effect that resulted in the highest scores on the gender-role inadequacy scale.

Note that because this is an ex post facto study, there is nothing in the data to establish causal relationships. Carroll cannot conclude that depression and feelings of gender-role inadequacy are a consequence of an infertility problem or of being the responsible party in a couple's fertility problem. The direction of causality, after all, might be reversed: people who are depressed may have a psychogenic block that inhibits fertility. Or, the results could reflect the effects of some other characteristics that differentiate the four groups. Statistical significance tells us nothing about whether there is a cause-and-effect relationship; it tells us that there is a high probability that the relation exists in the population.

2. Here is a brief summary of another fictitious study. Read the summary and then respond to the questions that follow.

Bentley (1996) hypothesized that infants' sleeping problems were related to various conditions and experiences during their birth. Fifty infants aged 3 to 6 months were diagnosed as having severe sleep disturbance problems. A group of 50 infants aged 3 to 6 months who had normal sleeping patterns was used as the comparison group. Bentley obtained the hospital records for all 100 children. The two groups were compared in terms of the following variables: amount of anesthesia administered during labor and delivery (none, small amount, large amount); length of time in labor (number of hours and minutes); type of delivery (cesarean or vaginal); birth weight (in grams); and Apgar scores at 3 minutes (scores from 1 to 10). Bentley found that the sleep disturbance group had had significantly longer time in labor than the comparison group. The groups were comparable in terms of the other variables.

Review and critique this research effort. Suggest alternative measurement approaches. To assist you in your critique, here are some guiding questions:
a. How many variables were measured in this study?
b. For each variable, identify the level of measurement that was used.
c. For each variable, indicate whether the measurement could have been made at a higher level of measurement than the level that was used. If yes, specify how you might measure the variable to obtain a higher level measure.
d. For two of the variables, write out operational definitions that clearly indicate the rules of measurement for those variables.

3. Below are several suggested research articles. Read one of these articles, paying special attention to the ways in which the research variables were operationalized. Evaluate the researcher's measurement strategy, using parts a to d of Question D.2 as a guide.
- Bowman, J. M. (1994). Perception of surgical pain by nurses and patients. *Clinical Nursing Research, 3,* 69–76.
- Johnson, J. E. (1996). Social support and physical health in the rural elderly. *Applied Nursing Research, 9,* 61–66.
- Moore, S. M. (1996). CABG discharge information. *Clinical Nursing Research, 5,* 97–104.
- Yarcheski, A., & Knapp-Spooner, C. (1994). Stressors associated with coronary bypass surgery. *Clinical Nursing Research, 3,* 57–68.

4. Here is another brief summary of a fictitious study. Read the summary and then respond to the questions that follow.

> *Langevin (1996) hypothesized that patients with a high degree of physical mobility would describe themselves as being healthier than patients with less physical mobility. To test this hypothesis, 120 male patients in a Veterans Administration hospital were asked to rate themselves on a five-point scale regarding their current physical health (1 = very unhealthy and 5 = very healthy) and to predict the number of days that they would be hospitalized. Forty of these patients had been categorized as "of limited mobility," another 40 were classified as "of moderate mobility," and the remaining 40 were described as "of high mobility." Langevin reported his descriptive findings as follows:*
>
> > *The self-ratings of physical health were fairly normally distributed for the sample as a whole: 42% rated themselves as neither healthy nor unhealthy; 7% and 21% described themselves as "very healthy" or "somewhat healthy," respectively. At the other extreme, 6% said they were "very unhealthy," and 24% said "somewhat unhealthy." The three groups differed in this regard, however. In the high-mobility group, a full 45% said they were either "very" or "somewhat healthy," whereas only 30% of the moderate-mobility and 15% of the low-mobility groups said this. For the entire sample, the mean predicted length of stay was 14.1 days. The median length, however, was only 12.5 days. For the three groups, the means and standard deviations with respect to predicted length of stay in hospital were as follows:*

	Mean	**Standard Deviation**
High Mobility	7.1	3.2
Moderate Mobility	11.9	4.5
Low Mobility	23.3	7.4

> > *In this sample of patients, the correlation between predicted length of stay in hospital and the health rating was .56.*

Review and critique this study, particularly with respect to the statistical analysis. To assist you in this critique, here are some guiding questions:

a. Which of the following types of descriptive statistical methods were used in this example?

- Frequency distribution
- Measure of central tendency
- Measure of variability
- Contingency table
- Correlation

b. Comment on the appropriateness of each statistic reported in the example. Is the statistic appropriate given the level of measurement of the variable? Does the statistic throw away information? Is the statistic the most stable statistic possible?

c. Identify two or three statistics that were not reported by the researcher that could have been reported given the data that were collected. Evaluate the extent to which the absence of this information weakened (or streamlined) the report of the results.

d. Discuss the meaning of the means and standard deviations in this example.

5. Below are several suggested research articles. Skim one (or more) of these articles and respond to parts a to d of Question D.4 in terms of the actual research study. (At this point, ignore the references to tests of statistical significance, which are covered in subsequent exercises.)

- Bostrom, J., Caldwell, J., McGuire, K., & Everson, D. (1996). Telephone follow-up after discharge from the hospital: Does it make a difference? *Applied Nursing Research, 9,* 47–52.
- Evans, B. D., & Rogers, A. E. (1994). 24-hour sleep/wake patterns in healthy elderly persons. *Applied Nursing Research, 7,* 75–83.
- Trepanier, M., Niday, P., Davies, B., Sprague, A., Nimrod, C., Dulberg, C., & Watters, N. (1996). Evaluation of a fetal monitoring education program. *Journal of Obstetric, Gynecologic, and Neonatal Nursing, 25,* 137–144.
- Ward, S. E., Berry, P. E., & Misiewicz, H. (1996). Concerns about analgesics among patients and family caregivers in a hospice setting. *Research in Nursing & Health, 19,* 205–211.

6. Below is another brief summary of a fictitious study. Read the summary and then respond to the questions that follow.

Kuhara (1997) investigated whether taste acuity declines with age, using a cross-sectional design. Eighty subjects were given a taste acuity test in which they were asked to indicate, for 25 substances, whether the taste was salty, sweet, bitter, or sour. The substances were presented in randomized order. Each person had five scores: four scores corresponding to the correct identification of the substances in the four taste categories, and one total score. Twenty subjects from each of the following age groups were tested: 31 to 40, 41 to 50, 51 to 60, and 61 to 70 years. It was hypothesized that taste acuity would decline with age, both overall and for all four subcategories of taste. The mean test scores for the four groups on all five outcomes measures appear below, together with information on the statistical tests performed.

	Age Group				F	df	p
	31–40	41–50	51–60	61–70			
Salty test	6.3	5.8	5.7	5.4	3.5	3,76	<.05
Sweet test	5.0	5.0	5.4	5.2	1.2	3,76	>.05
Bitter test	4.0	4.1	3.7	3.3	2.6	3,76	>.05
Sour test	1.9	2.0	2.0	2.1	0.8	3,76	>.05
Overall test	17.2	16.9	16.8	16.0	2.4	3,76	>.05

> *Kuhara concluded that her hypothesis was only partially supported by the data.*

Review and critique the above study. Suggest possible alternatives for handling the analysis of the data. To assist you in your critique, here are some guiding questions.

a. For each of the variables, indicate the actual level of measurement as used, then indicate the highest possible level of measurement for each. Is there a discrepancy? If so, can you think of a justification for it?

b. What statistical test was used to analyze the data? Did the researcher use the appropriate statistical test? If not, what statistical test do you think would be more suitable?

c. Are the degrees of freedom as presented correct?

d. Which of the results is statistically significant—that is, which hypothesis was supported by the data? Describe the meaning of each of the statistical tests.

7. Below are several suggested research articles. Skim one (or more) of these articles and respond to parts a to d of Question D.6 in terms of the actual research study.

- Bruce, S. L., & Grove, S. K. (1994). The effect of a coronary artery risk evaluation program on serum lipid values and cardiovascular risk levels. *Applied Nursing Research, 7,* 67–74.

- Gulick, E. E. (1994). Social support among persons with multiple sclerosis. *Research in Nursing & Health, 17,* 195–206.

- Northouse, L. L., Laten, D., & Reddy, P. (1995). Adjustment of women and their husbands to recurrent breast cancer. *Research in Nursing & Health, 18,* 515–524.

- Oertwich, P. A., Kindschuh, A. M., & Bergstrom, N. (1996). The effects of small shifts in body weight on blood flow and interface pressure. *Research in Nursing & Health, 18,* 481–488.

- Ronen, T., & Abraham, Y. (1996). Retention control training in the treatment of younger versus older enuretic children. *Nursing Research, 45,* 78–81.

◪ E. SPECIAL PROJECTS

1. Fictitious data from 24 nurses for six variables are presented below. Compute and present 5 to 10 different descriptive statistics that you think would best summarize this information.

Subject No.	Shift[a]	Anxiety Scores[b]	Supervisor's Performance Rating[c]	No. of Years of Experience	Marital Status[d]	Job Satisfaction Score[e]
1	1	10	4	5	2	4
2	1	13	4	2	2	5
3	1	8	2	1	1	3
4	1	4	7	10	1	3
5	1	6	9	12	1	4
6	1	9	8	7	1	2
7	1	12	6	8	2	4
8	1	5	4	2	1	5
9	2	10	5	4	2	1
10	2	14	6	1	2	4
11	2	8	5	3	1	5
12	2	15	8	2	2	2
13	2	11	8	7	2	3
14	2	14	7	9	1	1
15	2	1	5	3	2	2
16	2	8	8	6	1	3
17	3	3	7	19	2	4
18	3	7	4	7	1	1
19	3	19	5	1	2	2
20	3	5	6	11	1	1
21	3	8	3	2	1	3
22	3	10	4	5	2	2
23	3	13	6	6	2	1
24	3	14	5	3	1	2

[a]1 = day; 2 = evening; 3 = night

[b]Scores are from a low of 0 to a high of 20, 20 = most anxious

[c]Ratings are from 1 = poor to 9 = excellent

[d]1 = married; 2 = not married

[e]Scores are from low of 1 to high of 5; 5 = most satisfied

2. Ask 20 friends, classmates, or colleagues the following three questions:
- How many brothers and sisters do you have?
- How many children do you expect to have in total?
- Would you describe your family during your childhood as "very close," "fairly close," or "not very close"?

When you have gathered your data, calculate and present several statistics that describe the information you obtained.

3. Below is a list of variables. Assume that you have data from 500 nurses on these variables. Develop two or three hypotheses regarding the relationships among these variables and indicate what statistical tests you would use to test your hypotheses.
- Number of years of nursing experience
- Type of employment setting (hospital, nursing school, public school system, etc.)
- Salary
- Marital status
- Job satisfaction ("dissatisfied," "neither dissatisfied nor satisfied," or "satisfied")
- Number of children under age 18
- Gender

4. Design and describe a study in which you would use both factor analysis and discriminant function analysis.

Chapter 12
The Analysis of Qualitative Data

◣ A. MATCHING EXERCISES

1. Match each descriptive statement from Set B with one of the types of analytic strategy from Set A. Indicate the letter corresponding to your response next to each item in Set B.

Set A

a. Quasi-statistical style
b. Template analysis style
c. Editing analysis style
d. Immersion/crystallization style

Set B   *Responses*

1. Approach is sometimes referred to as manifest content analysis   _____
2. Researcher becomes totally involved in and reflective of the data _____
3. Grounded theory approach typically adopts this analytic style   _____
4. Fits the data to a preestablished codebook   _____
5. Type of style most likely to be adopted by ethnographers   _____
6. Researcher develops an analysis guide that is used to sort and
   interpret the data   _____

◣ B. COMPLETION EXERCISES

Write the words or phrases that correctly complete the sentences below.

1. Data collection and data analysis typically occur _____
   _____ in qualitative studies, not as separate phases.

2. The four processes that play a role in qualitative analysis are _____
   _____, _____,
   _____, and _____
   _____.

3. The main task in organizing qualitative data involves the development of a method of _____ and _____ _____ the data.

4. The process of breaking down the data, examining them, and comparing them to other segments is referred to as _____.

5. In a grounded theory study, the initial phase of coding is referred to as _____.

6. A _____ is a physical file that is organized to contain all material relating to a topic area.

7. Traditional methods of organizing qualitative data are being replaced by _____.

8. The analysis of qualitative data generally begins with a search for _____.

9. The use of _____ involves an accounting of the frequency with which certain themes and relationships are supported by the data.

10. _____ is a method that involves an iterative approach to testing research hypotheses with qualitative data.

11. Another name for level II coding in the grounded theory approach is _____.

12. Level III coding results in a description of a _____ _____ (BSP).

▨ C. STUDY QUESTIONS

1. Define the following terms. Use the textbook to compare your definition with the definition in Chapter 12 or in the Glossary.

   a. Qualitative analysis: _____ _____

   b. Categorization scheme: _____ _____

   c. Template: _____ _____

   d. Theme: _____ _____

   e. Memos: _____ _____

    f. Selective coding: _____

    _____

    g. Core category: _____

    _____

2. For each of the problem statements below, indicate whether you think a researcher should collect primarily qualitative or quantitative data.

    a. How do victims of AIDS cope with the discovery of their illness?

    _____

    _____

    b. What important dimensions of nursing practice differ in developed and underdeveloped countries?

    _____

    _____

    c. What is the effect of therapeutic touch on patient well-being?

    _____

    _____

    d. Do nurse practitioners and physicians differ in the performance of triage functions?

    _____

    _____

    e. Is a patient's length of stay in hospital related to the quality or quantity of his or her social supports?

    _____

    _____

    f. How does the typical American feel about such new reproductive technologies as in vitro fertilization?

    _____

    _____

    g. By what processes do women make decisions about having an amniocentesis?

    _____

    _____

    h. What are the psychological sequelae of having an organ transplant?

    _____

    _____

      i. What factors are most predictive of a woman giving birth to a very low-birth-weight infant?

_____

_____

      j. What effects does caffeine have on gastrointestinal motility?

_____

_____

3. In the following grounded theory study, identify what the researcher focused on as the basic social process: Reutter, L. I., & Northcott, H. C., (1994). Achieving a sense of control in a context of uncertainty: Nurses and AIDS. *Qualitative Health Research, 4,* 51–71.

4. A category scheme for coding interviews with recently divorced women follows:

  1. Divorce-related issues
    a. Adjustment to divorce
    b. Divorce-induced problems
    c. Advantages of divorce
  2. General psychologic state
    a. Before divorce
    b. During divorce
    c. Current
  3. Physical health
    a. Before divorce
    b. During divorce
    c. Current
  4. Relationship with children
    a. General quality
    b. Communication
    c. Shared activities
    d. Structure of relationship
  5. Parenting
    a. Discipline and childrearing
    b. Feelings about parenthood
    c. Feelings about single parenthood
  6. Friendships/social participation
    a. Dating and marriage
    b. Friendships
    c. Social groups, leisure
    d. Social support
  7. Employment/education
    a. Employment experiences
    b. Educational experiences

     c. Job and career goals
     d. Educational goals
  8. Workload
     a. Coping with workload
     b. Schedule
     c. Child care arrangements
  9. Finances

Read the following excerpt, taken from a real interview. Use the coding scheme to code the topics discussed in this excerpt.

> *I think raising children is so much easier without the father around. There isn't two people conflicting back and forth. You know, like. . . . like you discipline them during the day. They do something wrong, you're not saying, "When Daddy gets home, you're going to get a spanking." You know you do that. The kids get a spanking right then and there. But when two people live together, they have their ways of raising and you have your ways of raising the children and it's so hard for two people to raise children. It's so much easier for one person. The only reason a male would be around is financial-wise. But me and the kids are happier now, and we get along with each other better, cause like there isn't this competitive thing. My husband always wanted all the attention around here.*

▨ D. APPLICATION EXERCISES

1. Below is a brief description of the data analysis in a fictitious qualitative study, followed by a critique. Do you agree with this critique? Can you add other comments relevant to the data analysis in this study? (Box 12-1 offers some guiding questions.)

> ***Fictitious Study.*** *Wardlaw (1996) was interested in learning about the health policies and health environments of child care centers. She began her study by spending a week in an urban day care center that provided child care services to children aged 10 weeks to preschool-age. The purpose of this preliminary step was to ascertain likely sources of information and to familiarize herself with the routine of child care environments.*
>
> *The data for the study were collected through unstructured interviews with child care staff, through observation of activities during normal operating hours, and through the gathering of formal health policy statements from the administrators of the centers. The interviews with the staff focused*

on how staff handled illnesses among the children, what the patterns of illnesses were, how parents were notified in the case of a midday illness, to what extent medications were administered by the staff, what the staff did to minimize contagion, and how the staff interpreted center policies relating to the admission of unwell children. Data were collected from 10 child care centers that served 25 or more children whose ages ranged from infant to preschool-age. A total of 68 staff interviews were completed.

Wardlaw's field notes from the observations and the interviews were transcribed and coded according to a coding scheme that evolved during the actual collection of data. Three major themes emerged from the data analysis. These were labeled uncertainty, conflict, and frustration. The types of evidence that gave rise to the uncertainty category included statements made by staff, such as: "I'm really not a very good judge of just where to draw the line in deciding whether to keep a child here or send her home"; "I can't really remember what our health policies say on that"; and "I don't really know what the major health problems are among our kids—when they're absent, I just have one less kid to worry about."

Evidence of the conflict dimension included the researcher's observation that staff and parents sometimes had disagreements about whether a child was not well enough to attend. Also, staff made such statements as: "Health is a problem in child care centers because, on the one hand, allowing a sick kid to attend means that we'll have a lot of sick kids, but on the other hand, it's really tough on parents when their child care arrangements fall apart."

The category of frustration emerged from such statements as: "It's difficult to plan activities because absenteeism for health reasons is such a problem right now" and "I can't seem to get the kids interested in thinking about good health or good nutrition—their parents are just as bad."

Wardlaw analyzed the data herself but shared preliminary results of her analyses with one of the directors of a child care center, who concurred with the thematic analysis. Wardlaw's analysis showed that centers that had a formal arrangement with a health care provider were less likely to have staff who were uncertain. Conflict was a fairly universal theme but appeared to be more prevalent among those centers that served predominantly low-income families. Frustration was most likely to be observed and expressed among staff caring for older children.

Critique. Given Wardlaw's broad area of interest in health issues within child care centers, it seems appropriate that she conducted an in-depth, multi-faceted, qualitative study. The use of three complementary sources of data strengthened her study because it provided an opportunity for validating findings. At least from the brief description presented, however, it does not appear that these data sources were fully exploited. For example, no use appears to have been made of the written policy statements.

It appears that the author did little to validate the subjective thematic analysis. The analysis would have been greatly strengthened if Wardlaw had involved another investigator in the coding and analysis, if she had systematically searched for contrary evidence regarding the important themes, or if there had been an iterative approach in the analysis to check emerging themes against the data. Although it is laudable that Wardlaw invited comments from one of the child care center's directors, this procedure by itself provided a relatively weak form of validation.

The true validity of Wardlaw's thematic analysis is difficult to evaluate thoroughly without actually inspecting the data, but the brief description does not provide persuasive evidence that the analysis was thorough and unbiased. The data sources should have yielded a wealth of information about various aspects of the health policies and practices of the day care centers. Yet all three themes focus on the staff's feelings, and in all three cases these are negative feelings. What about their actions? What about their levels of competence in dealing with health issues? What about their sensitivity to the needs of their clients? It would appear that several of the excerpts included in support of Wardlaw's thematic analysis could have been conceptualized in a different way, suggesting that perhaps Wardlaw had some preconceived notions about what the unstructured interviews and observations would yield. It is possible that a reconceptualization (i.e., a thematic analysis of the same materials by a different investigator) could completely alter our impression of the health practices and policies of child care centers.

2. Here is a brief summary of another fictitious qualitative study. Read the summary and then respond to the questions that follow.

Crootof (1996) studied the phenomenon of "being on precautions" from the perspective of hospitalized adults. She began her study by spending 2 days on the hospital units where the data would be collected. The 2 days were spent familiarizing herself with the units, learning how best to collect the data, determining where she could position herself in an unobtrusive manner, and establishing a trusting relationship with the nursing staff.

The data for the study were collected using the techniques of observation and unstructured interviewing. Crootof selectively sampled all times of the day and all days of the week in 2-hour segments to make her observations. The time schedule began on a Monday morning at 7 AM and continued until 9 AM. On Tuesday, the observation time became 9 AM until 11 AM. Observations continued around the clock on consecutive days until no new information was being collected. Crootof positioned herself either directly outside the door to the patient's room or sat in the patient's room to make her observations. Observations included any activity or interaction between the patient and hospital staff or between the patient and herself.

The unstructured interviewing process consisted of asking patients to clarify why they were doing certain things and what they liked or disliked about the hospital experience.

Crootof recorded the observations and data from the interviews in a log immediately after each 2-hour observation segment. All data were recorded in chronologic order. In addition to the above, Crootof also recorded any feelings she had during the observation experience. As time progressed, she reread her field notes after every 4 hours of observation. As commonalities began to emerge from the data, she developed another section to her log according to similarity of content and referenced the daily log notes according to commonalities. Crootof continued making observations until she believed she had a "feel for the data," and additional observations or interactions provided only redundant information. A total of four patients were observed.

Themes that emerged from the data were labeled "avoidance," "devaluation as a person," and "loneliness." Evidence for the avoidance perspective came from patient comments during informal conversations with the researcher and the observational field notes. The evidence included statements such as, "Nurses seldom come into the room because they have to put all that (pointing to precaution gowns) stuff on"; "Look, she (the cleaning woman) won't come in the room. She's afraid of me"; "Did you see that? Only my doctor would touch me. The rest were afraid to touch me." Observational field notes con-

tained several notations of nurses coming to the door of the room asking, "Do you want anything?" but not entering the room.

The theme "loneliness" was developed from observations of patients occasionally putting the call light on to find out what time it was or how long until lunch, or asking about a noise they had heard. Comments that conveyed the same feeling of loneliness were "Being confined in this room is like being in jail"; "I can't wait to get out of here and have dinner with my friends"; and "The hours seem endless here."

Review and critique this study. Suggest alternative ways of collecting and analyzing the data for the research problem. To assist you in your critique, consider the following guiding questions, as well as the questions in Box 12-1 of the text.

a. Which of the four qualitative analysis styles did the researcher use?
b. How did the researcher handle the concept of saturation? Could you recommend any improvements?
c. What types of validation procedures did the researcher use? Can you suggest additional procedures that might have improved the study?
d. Comment on the thematic categories that emerged from the data. Do they seem to reflect accurately the data that were collected? Would you have developed different ones?

3. Below are several suggested research articles. Skim one of these articles and respond to relevant parts of Question D.2 in terms of an actual research study.
- Admi, H. (1996). Growing up with a chronic health condition: A model of an ordinary lifestyle. *Qualitative Health Research, 6,* 163–183.
- Badger, T. A. (1996). Family members' experiences living with members with depression. *Western Journal of Nursing Research, 18,* 149–171.
- Johnson, R. A. (1996). The meaning of relocation among elderly religious sisters. *Western Journal of Nursing Research, 18,* 172–185.
- Saveman, B.I., Hallberg, I. R., & Norberg, A. (1996). Narratives by district nurses about elder abuse within families. *Clinical Nursing Research, 5,* 220-236.

◩ E. SPECIAL PROJECTS

1. Get 10 or so people to write one or two paragraphs on their concerns about rising health care costs. Perform a thematic analysis of these paragraphs.
2. Develop two or three research questions that you think might lend themselves to a qualitative study.
3. Read one of the studies listed in the Suggested Readings of Chapter 12. Generate several hypotheses based on the reported findings.

Critical Appraisal and Utilization of Nursing Research

PART VI

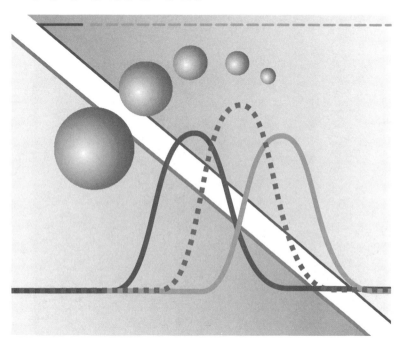

Chapter 13
Critiquing Research Reports

▨ A. MATCHING EXERCISES

1. Match each of the questions in Set B with the research decision for quantitative studies that is being evaluated, as listed in Set A. Indicate the letter(s) corresponding to your response next to each of the statements in Set B.

Set A

a. Evaluating the research design decisions
b. Evaluating the population and sampling plan
c. Evaluating the data collection procedures
d. Evaluating the analytic decisions

Set B   *Responses*

1. Were there a sufficient number of subjects?   _____
2. Was there evidence of adequate reliability and validity? _____
3. Would a more limited specification have controlled some
   extraneous variables not covered by the research design? _____
4. Would nonparametric tests have been more appropriate?   _____
5. Should a stratified design have been used?   _____
6. Were threats to internal validity adequately controlled? _____
7. Were the statistical tests appropriate, given the level of
   measurement of the variables?   _____
8. Were response set biases minimized?   _____
9. Was the comparison group equivalent to the experimental
   group?   _____
10. Should the data have been collected prospectively?   _____

2. Match each of the questions in Set B with the research decision for qualitative studies that is being evaluated, as listed in Set A. Indicate the letter(s) corresponding to your response next to each of the statements in Set B.

Set A

a. Evaluating the setting
b. Evaluating data sources and data quality
c. Evaluating the sampling plan
d. Evaluating the data analysis

Set B   *Responses*

1. Were triangulation procedures used as a method of validation?   _____
2. Were there a sufficient number of study participants to achieve saturation?   _____
3. Were constant comparison procedures appropriately used to refine relevant categories?   _____
4. Was the method of data collection appropriate and sufficient?   _____
5. Were participants asked to comment on the emerging themes?   _____
6. Did the study take place in an information-rich location?   _____
7. Were the study participants the best possible informants?   _____
8. Do the themes seem parsimonious, logical, and nonsuperficial?   _____

◨ B. COMPLETION EXERCISES

1. The first step in the interpretation of research findings involves an analysis of the _____ of the results, based on various types of evidence.

2. Interpretation of quantitative results is easiest when the results are consistent with the researcher's _____.

3. An important research precept is that correlation does not prove _____ _____.

4. Researchers should avoid the temptation of going beyond _____ _____.

5. Statistical significance does not necessarily mean that research results are _____.

6. The research process involves numerous methodologic _____ _____, each of which could affect the quality of the study.

7. A good critique should identify both _____ and _____ in a study.

8. An evaluation of the relevance of a study to some aspect of the nursing profession involves critiquing the _____ dimension of a research study.

9. An evaluation of the researcher's study design involves critiquing the _____ _____ dimension of a research study.

10. An evaluation of the way in which human subjects were treated involves critiquing the _____ dimension of a research study.

11. An evaluation of the sense the researcher tried to make of the results involves critiquing the _____ dimension of the research study.

12. An evaluation of the conciseness and organization of the research report involves critiquing the _____ dimension of the research study.

▨ C. STUDY QUESTIONS

1. Define the following terms. Use the textbook to compare your definitions with the definitions in Chapter 13 or in the Glossary.

a. Critique: _____
_____

b. Results: _____
_____

c. Interpretation of results: _____
_____

d. Unhypothesized results: _____
_____

e. Mixed results: _____
_____

2. Read the research report by Gretchen Randolph entitled "Therapeutic and physical touch: Physiological response to stressful stimuli," which appeared in the January 1984 issue of *Nursing Research* (volume 33, pages 33–36). None of the researcher's hypotheses were supported. Review and critique Randolph's interpretations of the findings and suggest some possible alternative explanations.

3. Below are several suggested research reports for studies in which the researcher obtained mixed results—that is, some hypotheses were supported and others were not. Review and critique the researcher's interpretation of the findings for one of these studies, and suggest possible alternatives.

- Blair, C. E. (1995). Combining behavior management and mutual goal setting to reduce physical dependency in nursing home residents. *Nursing Research, 44,* 160–165.
- Jadack, R. A., Hyde, J. S., & Keller, M. L. (1995). Gender knowledge about HIV, risky sexual behavior, and safer sex practices. *Research in Nursing & Health, 18,* 313–324.
- Miller, K. M., & Perry, P. A. (1990). Relaxation technique and postoperative pain in patients undergoing cardiac surgery. *Heart and Lung, 19,* 136–146.
- Naylor, M. D. (1990). Comprehensive discharge planning for hospitalized elderly: A pilot study. *Nursing Research, 39,* 156–161.

4. Read and critique one or more of the following research reports (or others in the nursing research literature). Apply the guidelines in Chapter 13 of the textbook to the article. Prepare two or three pages of "bullet points" that indicate the major strengths and weaknesses of the study.

Quantitative Studies

- Birenbaum, L. K., Stewart, B.J., & Phillips, D. S. (1996). Health status of bereaved parents. *Nursing Research, 45,* 105–109.
- Carty, E. M. (1996). Women's perceptions of fatigue during pregnancy and postpartum: The impact of length of stay in hospital. *Clinical Nursing Research, 5,* 67–80.
- Edberg, A., Hallberg, I. R., & Gustafson, L. (1996). Effects of clinical supervision on nurse-patient cooperation quality. *Clinical Nursing Research, 5,* 127–149.
- Heidrich, S. M. (1996). Mechanisms related to psychological well-being in older women with chronic illnesses: Age and disease comparisons. *Research in Nursing & Health, 19,* 225–235.
- Milligan, R. A., Flenniken, P. M., & Pugh, L. C. (1996). Positioning intervention to minimize fatigue in breastfeeding women. *Applied Nursing Research, 9,* 67-70.

Qualitative Studies

- Hinds, P. S., et al. (1996). Coming to terms: Parents' response to a first cancer recurrence in their child. *Nursing Research, 45,* 148–153.
- Quayhagen, M. P., & Quayhagen, M. (1996). Discovering life quality in coping with dementia. *Western Journal of Nursing Research, 18,* 120–135.
- Sebern, M. D. (1996). Explication of the construct of shared care and the prevention of pressure ulcers in home health care. *Research in Nursing & Health, 19,* 183–192.
- Woodgate, R., & Kristjanson, L. J. (1996). "My hurts": Hospitalized young children's perceptions of acute pain. *Qualitative Health Research, 6,* 184–201.
- Wurzbach, M. E. (1996). Long-term care nurses' ethical convictions about tube feeding. *Western Journal of Nursing Research, 18,* 63–76.

5. Read the following study and identify its major strengths and limitations:
   - Gilbert, D. A. (1993). Reciprocity of involvement activities in client-nurse interactions. *Western Journal of Nursing Research, 15,* 674–687.

   Now, read Weiss's commentary of Gilbert's study that immediately follows the report (pages 687–688). Do any of your comments overlap with those of Weiss? Do you agree or disagree with Weiss's comments?

▧ D. APPLICATION EXERCISES

1. Following is a fictitious research report and a critique of various aspects of the report. This example is designed to highlight features about the form and content of both a written report and a written evaluation of the study's worth. To economize on space, the report is rather brief, but it incorporates the essential elements for a meaningful appraisal.

   Read the report and critique, and then determine whether you agree with the critique. Can you add other comments relevant to a critical appraisal of the study?

The Report: *The Role of Health Care Providers in Teenage Pregnancy* by Phyllis Nelson, 1992

Background

Of the 20 million teenagers living in the United States today, about one in five is sexually active by age 14; more than half have had sexual intercourse by age 19 (Kelman and Saner, 1989).* Despite increased availability of contraceptives, the number of teenage pregnancies has risen at an alarming rate

---

*All references in this example are fictitious, although most of the information in this fictitious literature review is based on real studies and is therefore reasonably accurate.

over the past two decades. Over one million girls under age 20 become pregnant each year and, of these, about 500,000 become teenaged mothers (U.S. Bureau of the Census, 1985).

Public concern regarding the teenage pregnancy epidemic stems not only from the rising number of involved teenagers but also from the extensive research that has documented the adverse consequences of early parenthood in the health arena. Pregnant teenagers have been found to receive less prenatal care (Tremain, 1992), to be more likely to develop toxemia (Schendley, 1981; Waters, 1989), to be more likely to experience prolonged labor (Curran, 1979), to be more likely to have low-birth-weight babies (Tremain, 1992; Beach, 1987), and to be more likely to have babies with low Apgar scores (Beach, 1987) than older mothers. The long-term consequences to the teenaged mothers themselves are also extremely bleak: teenaged mothers get less schooling, are more likely to be on public assistance, are likely to earn lower wages, and are more likely to get divorced if they marry than their peers who postpone parenthood (Jamail, 1989; North, 1982; Smithfield, 1979).

The one million teenagers who become pregnant each year are caught up in a tough emotional decision—to carry the pregnancy to term and keep the baby, to have an abortion, or to deliver the baby and surrender it for adoption. Despite the widely reported adverse consequences of young parenthood cited above, most young women today are opting for delivery and child-rearing, often out of wedlock (Jaffrey, 1988; Henderson, 1991).

The purpose of this study was to test the effect of a special intervention based in an outpatient clinic of a Chicago hospital on improving the health outcomes of a group of pregnant teenagers. Specifically, it was hypothesized that pregnant teenagers who were in the special program would receive more prenatal care, would be less likely to develop toxemia, would be less likely to have a low-birth-weight baby, would spend fewer hours in labor, would have babies with higher Apgar scores, and would be more likely to use a contraceptive at 6 months postpartum than pregnant teenagers not enrolled in the program.

The theoretical model on which this research was based is an ecologic model of personal behavior (Brandenburg, 1984). A schematic diagram of the ecologic model is presented in Figure 13-A. In this framework, the actions of the person are the focus of attention, but those actions are believed to be a function not only of the person's own characteristics, atti-

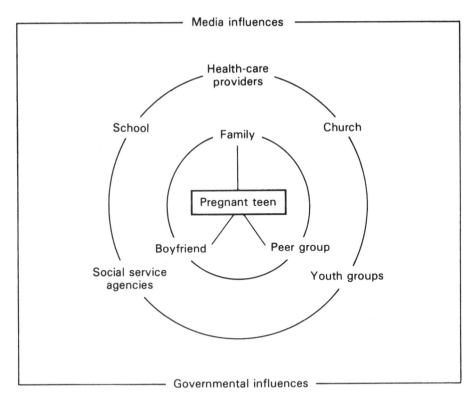

Figure 13-A. Model of ecologic contexts

*tudes, and abilities but also of other influences in their envi-
ronment. Environmental influences can be differentiated according to their proximal relationship with the target person.
Health care workers and institutions are, according to the
model, more distant influences than family, peers, and
boyfriends. Yet it is assumed that these less immediate forces
are real and can intervene to change the behaviors of the target person. Thus, it is hypothesized that pregnant teenagers
can be influenced by increased exposure to a health care team
providing a structured program of services designed to promote improved health outcomes.*

Methods

*A special program of services for pregnant teenagers was im-
plemented in the outpatient clinic of an inner-city public hospital in Chicago. The intervention involved nutrition education and counseling, parenting education, instruction on
prenatal health care, preparation for childbirth, and contraceptive counseling.*

All teenagers with a confirmed pregnancy attending the clinic were asked if they wanted to participate in the special program. The goal was to enroll 150 pregnant teenagers during the program's first year of operation. A total of 276 teenagers attending the clinic were invited to participate; of these, 59 had an abortion or miscarriage, and 108 declined to participate, yielding an experimental group sample of 109 girls.

To test the effectiveness of the special program, a comparison group of pregnant teenagers was needed. Another inner-city hospital agreed to cooperate in the study. Staff obtained information on the labor and delivery outcomes of the 120 teenagers who delivered at the comparison hospital, where no special teen-parent program was available. For both experimental group and comparison group subjects, a follow-up telephone interview was conducted 6 months postpartum to determine if the teenagers were using birth control.

The independent variable in this study was the teenager's program status: experimental group members participated in the special program, and comparison group members did not. The dependent variables were the teenagers' labor and delivery and postpartum contraceptive outcomes. The operational definitions of the dependent variables were as follows:

Prenatal care: Number of visits made to a physician or nurse during the pregnancy, exclusive of the visit for the pregnancy test
Toxemia: Presence versus absence of preeclamptic toxemia as diagnosed by a physician
Labor time: Number of hours elapsed from the first contractions until delivery of the baby, to the nearest half-hour
Low infant birth weight: Infant birth weights of less than 2500 g versus those of 2500 g or greater
Apgar score: Infant Apgar score (from 0 to 10) taken at 3 minutes after birth
Contraceptive use postpartum: Self-reported use of any form of birth control 6 months postpartum versus self-reported nonuse

The two groups were compared on these six outcome measures using t-tests and chi-squared tests.

Results

The teenagers in the sample were, on average, 17.6 years old at the time of delivery. The mean age was 17.1 in the experimental group and 18.0 in the comparison group.

By definition, all of the teenagers in the experimental group had received prenatal care. Two of the teenagers in the comparison group had no health care treatment before delivery. The distribution of visits for the two groups is presented in Figure 13-B. The experimental group had a higher mean number of prenatal visits than the comparison group, as shown in Table 13-A, but the difference was not statistically significant at the .05 level, using a t-test for independent groups.

In the sample as a whole, approximately 1 girl in 10 was diagnosed as having preeclamptic toxemia. The difference between the two groups was in the hypothesized direction, with 1.6% more of the comparison group teenagers developing this complication, but the difference was not significant using a chi-squared test.

The hours spent in labor ranged from 3.5 to 29.0 in the experimental group and from 4.5 to 33.5 in the comparison

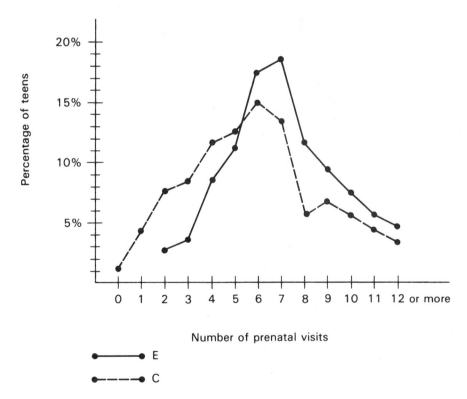

Figure 13-B. Frequency distribution of prenatal visits, by experimental versus comparison group. (*E,* experimental group; *C,* comparison group)

Table 13-A. Summary of Experimental and Comparison Group Differences

Outcome Variable	Group		Difference	Test Statistic
	Experimental ($n = 109$)	Comparison ($n = 120$)		
Mean number of prenatal visits	7.1	5.9	1.2	$t = 1.83$, $df = 227$, NS
Percentage with toxemia	10.1%	11.7%	−1.6%	$\chi^2 = 0.15$, $df = 1$, NS
Mean hours spent in labor	14.3	15.2	−.09	$t = 1.01$, $df = 227$, NS
Percentage with low-birth-weight baby	16.5%	20.9%	−4.4%	$\chi^2 = 0.71$, $df = 1$, NS
Mean Apgar score	7.3	6.7	.6	$t = 0.98$, $df = 227$, NS
Percentage adopting contraception post-partum	81.7%	62.5%	19.2%	$\chi^2 = 10.22$, $df = 1$, $p < .01$

group. On average, teenagers in the experimental group spent 14.3 hours in labor, compared with 15.2 for the comparison group teenagers. The difference was not statistically significant.

With regard to low-birth-weight babies, a total of 43 girls out of 229 in the sample gave birth to babies who weighed under 2500 grams (5.5 pounds).[†] More of the comparison group teenagers (20.9%) than experimental group teenagers (16.5%) had low-birth-weight babies, but, once again, the group difference was not significant.

The 3-minute Apgar score in the two groups was quite similar—7.3 for the experimental group and 6.7 for the comparison group. This small difference was nonsignificant.

Finally, the teenagers were compared with respect to their adoption of birth control 6 months after delivering their babies. For this variable, teenagers were coded as users of contraception if they were either using some method of birth control at the time of the follow-up interview or if they were nonusers but were sexually inactive (i.e., were using absti-

---

[†]All mothers gave birth to live infants; however, there were two neonatal deaths within 24 hours of birth in the comparison group.

nence to prevent a repeat pregnancy). The results of the chi-squared test showed that a significantly higher percentage of experimental group teenagers (81.7%) than comparison group teenagers (62.5%) were using birth control after delivery. This difference was significant beyond the .01 level.

Discussion

The results of this evaluation were disappointing, but not discouraging. There was only one outcome for which a significant difference was observed. The experimental program significantly increased the percentage of teenagers who used birth control after delivering their babies. Thus, one highly important result of participating in the program is that an early repeat pregnancy will be postponed. There is abundant research that has shown that repeat pregnancy among teenagers is especially damaging to their educational and occupational attainment and leads to particularly adverse labor and delivery outcomes in the higher-order births (Klugman, 1985; Jackson, 1978).

The experimental group had more prenatal care, but not significantly more. Perhaps part of the difficulty is that the program can only begin to deliver services once pregnancy has been diagnosed. If a teenager does not come in for a pregnancy test until her fourth or fifth month, this obviously puts an upper limit on the number of visits she will have; it also gives less time for her to eat properly, avoid smoking and drinking, and take other steps to enhance her health during pregnancy. Thus, one implication of this finding is that the program needs to do more to encourage early pregnancy screening. Perhaps a joint effort between the clinic personnel and school nurses in neighboring middle schools and high schools could be launched to publicize the need for a timely pregnancy test and to inform teenagers where such a test could be obtained. The two groups performed similarly with respect to the various labor and delivery outcomes chosen to evaluate the effectiveness of the new program. The issue of timeliness is again relevant here. The program may have been delivering services too late in the pregnancy for the instruction to have made much of an impact on the health of the mother and her child. This interpretation is supported, in part, by the fact that the one variable for which timeliness was not an issue (postpartum contraception) was, indeed, positively affected by program participation. Another possible implication is that the program itself should be made more pow-

erful, for example, by lengthening or adding to instructional sessions.

Given that the experimental and comparison group differences were all in the hypothesized direction, it is also tempting to criticize the sample size. A larger sample (which was originally planned) might have yielded some significant differences.

In summary, the experimental intervention is not without promise. A particularly exciting finding is that participation in the program resulted in better contraceptive use, which will presumably lower the incidence of repeat pregnancy. It would be interesting to follow these teenagers 2 years after delivery to see if the groups differ in the rates of repeat pregnancy. It appears that more needs to be done to get these teenagers into the program early in their pregnancies. Perhaps then the true effectiveness of the program would be demonstrated.

Critique of the Research Report

In the following discussion, we present some comments on various aspects of this research report. Students are urged to read the report and formulate their own opinions about its strengths and weaknesses before reading this critique. An evaluation of a study is necessarily partly subjective. Therefore, it should be expected that students might disagree with some of the points made below. Other students may have additional criticisms and comments. We believe, however, that most of the serious methodologic flaws of the study are highlighted in our critique.

Title

The title for the study is misleading. The research does *not* investigate the role of health care professionals in serving the needs of pregnant teenagers. A more appropriate title would be "Health-Related Outcomes of an Intervention for Pregnant Teenagers."

Background

The background section of this report consists of three distinct elements that can be analyzed separately: a literature review, statement of the problem, and a theoretical framework.

The literature review is relatively clearly written and well organized. It serves the important function of establishing a need for the experimental program by documenting the prevalence of teenage pregnancy and some of its adverse consequences. However, the literature review could be improved. First, an inspection of the citations suggests that the author is not as up-to-date on research relating to teenage pregnancy as she might have been. Most of the references are from the 1980s or even earlier, meaning that this literature review is over a decade old. Second, there is material in the literature review section that is not relevant and should be removed. For example, the paragraph on the options with which a pregnant teenager is faced (paragraph 3) is not germane to the research problem. A third and more critical flaw is what the review does *not* cover. Given the research problem, there are probably four main points that should be addressed in the review:

1. How widespread is teenage pregnancy and parenthood?
2. What are the social and health consequences of early child-bearing?
3. What has been done (especially by nurses) to address the problems associated with teenage parenthood?
4. How successful have other interventions been?

The review adequately handles the first question: the need for concern is established. The second question is covered in the review, but perhaps more depth and more recent research is needed here. The new study is based on an assumption of negative health outcomes in teenaged mothers. The author has strung together a series of references without giving the reader any clues about the reliability of the information. The author would have made her point more convincingly if she had added a sentence such as "For example, in a carefully executed prospective study involving nearly 8000 pregnant women, Beach (1987) found that young maternal age was significantly associated with higher rates of prematurity and other negative neonatal outcomes." The third and fourth points that should have been covered are totally absent from the review. Surely the author's experimental program does not represent the first attempt to address the needs of pregnant teenagers. How is Nelson's intervention different from or better than other interventions? What reason does she have to believe that such an intervention might be successful? Nelson has provided a rationale for addressing the problem but no rationale for the manner in which she has addressed it. If, in fact, there is little information about other interventions and their effectiveness in improving health outcomes, then the review should say so.

The problem statement and hypothesis were stated succinctly and clearly. The hypothesis is complex (there are multiple dependent variables) and directional (it predicts better outcomes among teenagers participating in the special program).

The third component of the background section of the report is the theoretical framework. In our opinion, the theoretical framework chosen does little to enhance the research. The hypothesis is not generated on the basis of the model, nor does the intervention itself grow out of the model. One gets the feeling that the model was slapped on as an afterthought to try to make the study seem more sophisticated or theoretical. Actually, if more thought had been given to this conceptual framework, it might have proved useful. According to this model, the most immediate and direct influences on a pregnant teenager are her family, friends, and sexual partner. One programmatic implication of this is that the intervention should involve one or more of these influences. For example, a workshop for the teenagers' parents could have been developed to reinforce the teenagers' need for adequate nutrition and prenatal care. A research hypothesis that could have been tested in the context of the model is that teenagers who are missing one of the direct influences would be especially susceptible to the influence of less proximal health care providers (*i.e.*, the program). For example, it might be hypothesized that pregnant teenagers who do not live with both parents have to depend on alternative sources of social support (such as health care personnel) during the pregnancy. Thus, it is not that the theoretical context selected is far-fetched but rather that it was not convincingly linked to the actual research problem. Perhaps an alternative theoretical context would have been better. Or perhaps the researcher simply should have been honest and admitted that her research was practical, not theoretical.

Methods

The design used to test the research hypothesis was a widely used, preexperimental design. Two groups, whose equivalence is assumed but not established, were compared on several outcome measures. The design is one that has serious problems because the preintervention comparability of the groups is unknown.

The most serious threat to the internal validity of the study is selection bias. Selection bias can work both ways to mask true treatment effects or to create the illusion of a program effect when none exists. This is because selection bias can be either positive (*i.e.*, the experimental group can be initially advantaged in relation to the comparison group) or negative (*i.e.*, the experimental group can have pretreatment disadvantages). In the current study, it is possible that the two hospitals served clients of different economic circumstances, for example. If the average income of the families of the experimental group teenagers was higher, then these teenagers would probably have a better opportunity for adequate prenatal nutrition than the comparison group teenagers. Or the comparison hospital might serve older teens, or a higher percentage of married teens, or a higher percentage of teens attending a special school-based program for pregnant students. None of these extraneous variables, which could affect the mothers' health, has been controlled.

Another way in which the design was vulnerable to selection bias is the high refusal rate in the experimental group. Of the 217 eligible teenagers, half declined to participate in the special program. We cannot assume that the 109 girls who participated were a random sample of the eligible girls. Again, biases could be either positive or negative. A positive selection bias would be created if, for example, the teenagers who were the most motivated to have a healthy pregnancy selected themselves into the experimental group. A negative selection bias would result if the teenagers from the most disadvantaged households or from families offering little support elected to participate in the program. In the comparison group, hospital records were used primarily to collect the data, so this self-selection problem could not occur (except for refusals to answer the contraceptive questions 6 months postpartum).

The researcher could have taken a number of steps to either control selection biases or, at the least, estimate their direction and magnitude. The following are among the most critical extraneous variables: social class and family income, age, race and ethnicity, parity, participation in another pregnant teenager program, marital status, and prepregnancy experience with contraception (for the postpartum contraception outcome). The researcher should have attempted to gather information on these variables from experimental group and comparison group teenagers *and* from eligible teenagers in the experimental hospital who declined to participate in the program. To the extent that these three groups were found to be similar on these variables, credibility in the internal validity of the study would be enhanced. If sizable differences were observed, the researcher would at least know or suspect the direction of the biases and could factor that information into her interpretation and conclusions.

Had the researcher gathered information on the extraneous variables, another possibility would have been to match experimental and comparison group subjects on one or two variables, such as family income and age. Matching is not an ideal method of controlling extraneous variables; for one thing, matching on two variables would not equate the two groups in terms of the other extraneous variables. However, matching is preferable to doing nothing.

So far we have focused our attention on the research design, but other aspects of the study are also problematic. Let us consider the decision the researcher made about the population. The target population is not explicitly defined by the researcher, but one can infer that the target population is pregnant girls under age 20 who carry their infants to delivery. The accessible population is pregnant teenagers from one area in Chicago. Is it reasonable to assume that the accessible population is representative of the target population? No, it is not. It is likely that the accessible population is quite different with regard to health care, family intactness, and many other characteristics. The researcher should have more clearly discussed exactly who was the target population of this research.

Nelson would have done well, in fact, to delimit the target population; had she done so, it might have been possible to control some of the extraneous variables discussed previously. For example, Nelson could have established eligibility criteria that excluded multigravidas, very young teenagers (*e.g.,* younger than age 15), or married teenagers. Such a specification would have limited the generalizability of the findings, but it would have enhanced the internal validity of the study because it probably would have increased the comparability of the experimental and comparison groups.

The sample was a sample of convenience, the least effective sampling design for a quantitative study. There is no way of knowing whether the sample represents the accessible and target populations. Although probability sampling probably was not feasible, the researcher might have improved her sampling design by using a quota sampling plan. For example, if the researcher knew that in the accessible population, half of the families received public assistance, then it might have been possible to enhance the representativeness of the samples by using a quota system to ensure that half of the research subjects came from welfare-dependent families.

Sample size is a difficult issue. Many of the reported results were in the hypothesized direction but were nonsignificant. When this is the case, the adequacy of the sample size is always suspect, as Nelson pointed out. Each group had approximately 100 subjects. In many cases, this sample size would be considered adequate, but in the current case, it is not. One of the difficulties in testing the effectiveness of new interventions is that, generally, the experimental group is not being compared with a no-treatment group. Although the comparison group in this example was not getting the special program services, it cannot be assumed that this group was getting no services at all. Some comparison group members may have had ample prenatal care during which the health care staff may have provided much of the same information as they taught in the special program. The point is not that the new program was not needed but rather that unless an intervention is extremely powerful and innovative, the incremental improvement will typically be rather small. When relatively small effects are anticipated, the sample must be very large for differences to be statistically significant. Although it is beyond the scope of this book to explain the power analysis calculations, it can be shown that to detect a significant difference between the two groups with respect, say, to the incidence of toxemia, a sample of more than 5000 pregnant teenagers would have been needed. Had the researcher done a power analysis before conducting the study, she might have realized the insufficiency of her sample for some of the outcomes and might have developed a different sampling plan or identified different dependent variables.

The third major methodologic decision concerns the measurement of the research variables. For the most part, the researcher did a good job in selecting objective, reliable, and valid outcome measures. Also, her operational definitions were clearly worded and unambiguous. Two comments are in order, however. First, it might have been better to operationalize two of the variables differently. Infant birth weight might have been more sensitively measured as actual weight (a ratio-level measurement) or as a three-level ordinal variable (<1500 g; >1500 but <2500 g; and >2500 g) instead of as a dichotomous variable. The contraceptive variable could also have been measured differently to yield a more sensitive (*i.e.,* more discriminating) measure. Rather than measuring contraceptive use as a dichotomy, Nelson could have created an ordinal scale based on either frequency of use (*e.g.,* 0%, 1% to 25%, 26% to 50%, 51% to 75%, and 76% to 100% of the time) or on the effectiveness of the *type* of birth control used.

A second consideration is whether the outcome variables adequately captured the effects of program activities. It might have been easier, with the small sample of 229 teenagers, and more directly relevant, to capture group differences in, say, dietary practices during pregnancy than in infant birth weight. None of the outcome variables measured the effects of parenting education. In other words, the researcher could have added more direct measures of the effects of the special program.

One other point about the methods should be made, and that relates to ethical considerations. The article does not specifically say that subjects were asked for their informed consent, but that does not necessarily mean that no written consent was obtained. It is quite likely that the experimental group subjects, when asked to volunteer for the special program, were advised about their participation in the study and asked to sign a consent form. But what about the control group subjects? The article implies that comparison group members were given no opportunity to decline participation and were not aware of having their birth outcomes used as data in the research. In some cases, this procedure is acceptable. For example, a hospital or clinic might agree to release patient information without the patients' consent if the release of such information is done anonymously—that is, if it can be provided in such a way that even the researcher does not know the identity of the patients. In the current study, however, it is clear that the names of the comparison subjects *were* given to the researcher, because she had to contact the comparison group at 6 months postpartum to determine their contraceptive practices. Thus, this study does not appear to have adequately safeguarded the rights of the comparison group subjects.

In summary, the researcher appears not to have adhered to ethical procedures, and she also failed to give the new program a fair test. Nelson should have taken a number of steps to control extraneous variables and should have attempted to get a larger sample (even if this meant waiting for additional subjects to enroll in the program). In addition to concerns about the internal validity of the study, its generalizability is also questionable.

Results

Nelson did a good job of presenting the results of the study. The presentation was straightforward and succinct and was enhanced by the inclusion of a good table and figures. The style of this section was also appropriate: it was written objectively and was well organized.

The statistical analyses were also reasonably well done. The descriptive statistics (means and percentages) were appropriate for the level of measurement of the variables. The author did not, however, provide any information about the variability of the measures, except for noting the range for the "time spent in labor" variable. Figure 13-B suggests that the two groups did differ in variability: the comparison group was more heterogeneous than the experimental group with regard to prenatal care received.

The two types of inferential statistics used (the *t*-test and chi-squared test) were also appropriate, given the levels of measurement of the outcome variables. The results of these tests were efficiently presented in a single table. It should be noted that there are more powerful statistics available that could have been used to control extraneous variables (*e.g.,* analysis of covariance), but in the current study, it appears that the only extraneous variable that could have been controlled through statistical procedures was the subjects' ages because no data were apparently collected on other extraneous variables (social class, ethnicity, parity, and so on).

Discussion

Nelson's discussion section fails almost entirely to take the study's limitations into account in interpreting the data. The one exception is her acknowledgment that the sample size was too small. She seems unconcerned about the many threats to the internal or external validity of her research.

Nelson lays almost all the blame for the nonsignificant findings on the program rather than on the research methods. She thinks that two aspects of the program should be changed: (1) recruitment of teenagers into the program earlier in their pregnancies and (2) strengthening program services. Both recommendations might be worth pursuing, but there is little in the data to suggest these modifications. With nonsignificant results such as those that predominated in this study, there are two possibilities to consider: (1) the results are accurate—that is, the program is not effective for those outcomes examined (though it might be effective for other measures), and (2) the results are false—that is, the existing program is effective for the outcomes examined, but the tests failed to demonstrate it. Nelson concluded that the first possibility was correct and therefore recommended that the program be changed. Equally plausible is the possibility that the study methods were too weak to demonstrate the program's true effects.

We do not have enough information about the characteristics of the sample to conclude with certainty that there were substantial selection biases. We do, however, have a clue that selection biases were operative in a direction that would make the program look less effective than it actually is. Nelson noted in the beginning of the Results section that the average age of the teenagers in the experimental group was 17.1, compared with 18.0 in the comparison group. Age is inversely related to positive labor and delivery outcomes, indeed, that is the basis for having a special program for teenaged mothers. Therefore, the experimental group's performance on the outcome measures was possibly depressed by the youth of that group. Had the two groups been equivalent in terms of age, the group differences might have been larger and could have reached levels of statistical significance. Other uncontrolled pretreatment differences also could have masked true treatment effects.

For the one significant outcome, we cannot rule out the possibility that a Type I error was made—that is, that the null hypothesis was in fact true. Again, selection biases could have been operative. The experimental group might have contained many more girls who had preprogram experience with contraception; it might have contained more highly motivated teenagers, or more single teenagers, or more teenagers who had already had multiple pregnancies than the comparison group. There simply is no way of knowing whether the significant outcome reflects true program effectiveness or merely initial group differences.

Aside from Nelson's disregard for the problems of internal validity, the author definitely overstepped the bounds of scholarly speculation by reading too much into her data. She unquestionably assumed that the program *caused* contraceptive improvements: "the experimental program significantly increased the percentage of teenagers who used birth control. . . ." Worse yet, she went on to conclude that repeat pregnancies will be postponed in the experimental group, although she does not know whether the teenagers used an effective contraception, whether they used it all the time, or whether they used it correctly.

As another example of going beyond the data, Nelson became overly invested in her notion that teenagers need greater and earlier exposure to the program. It is not that her hypothesis has no merit—the problem is that she builds an elaborate rationale for program changes with no apparent empirical support. She probably had information on when in the pregnancy the teenagers entered the program, but that information was not shared with readers. Her argument about the need for more publicity on early screening would have had more clout if she had reported that most teenagers entered the program during the fourth month of their pregnancies or later. Additionally, she could have marshalled more evidence in support of her proposal if she had been able to show that earlier entry in the program was associated with better health outcomes. For example, she could have compared the outcomes of teenagers entering the program in the first, second, and third trimesters of their pregnancies.

In conclusion, the study has several attractive features. As Nelson noted, there is some reason to be cautiously optimistic that the program *could* have some beneficial effects. However, the existing study is too seriously flawed to reach any conclusions, even tentatively. A replication with improved research methods clearly is needed to solve the research problem.

2. At the end of this Study Guide, in Part VII, are two actual research reports, one for a quantitative study and the other for a qualitative study. Read one or both of these reports and prepare a three- to five-page critique summarizing the major strengths and weaknesses of the study.

◪ E. SPECIAL PROJECTS

1. Rewrite Nelson's report (Exercise D.1), using some of the suggestions from the critique or from classroom discussions.

2. Prepare a list of 10 critical questions that would need to be addressed in a critique of the methodological dimensions of a quantitative study. Select a recent research report for a quantitative study and apply those questions to it.

3. Prepare a list of the 10 critical questions that would need to be addressed in a critique of the methodological dimensions of a qualitative study. Select a recent research report for a quantitative study and apply those questions to it.

Chapter 14
Utilization of Nursing Research

A. MATCHING EXERCISES

1. Match each of the strategies from Set B with one of the roles indicated in Set A. Indicate the letters corresponding to your response next to each of the strategies in Set B.

Set A

a. Nurse researchers
b. Practicing nurses/nursing students
c. Nursing administrators

Set B	***Responses***
1. Become involved in a journal club	______
2. Perform replications	______
3. Offer resources for utilization projects	______
4. Disseminate findings	______
5. Specify clinical implications of findings	______
6. Read research reports critically	______
7. Foster intellectual curiosity in the work environment	______
8. Provide a forum for communication between clinicians and researchers	______
9. Expect evidence that a procedure is effective	______
10. Attend nursing conferences and research sessions	______

B. COMPLETION EXERCISES

Write the words or phrases that correctly complete the sentences below.

1. ______________________________ refers to the use of some aspect of a scientific investigation in an application unrelated to the original research.
2. There is considerable concern about the ______________________________ between knowledge production and knowledge utilization.

3. The most well-known nursing research utilization project, conducted in Michigan, is the _____ Project.

4. An early regional collaborative utilization project was the _____ _____ Project.

5. For research results to be believable, study findings must be _____ _____ in several different settings.

6. The three broad classes of criteria for research utilization are clinical relevance, scientific merit, and _____.

7. The issue of _____ concerns whether it makes sense to implement an innovation in a new practice setting.

8. A cost/benefit ratio assessment should consider not only the net cost and gain of implementing an innovation but also _____.

▨ C. STUDY QUESTIONS

1. Define the following terms. Use the textbook to compare your definition with the definition in Chapter 14 or in the Glossary.

a. Instrumental utilization: _____ _____

b. Conceptual utilization: _____ _____

c. Knowledge creep: _____ _____

d. Decision accretion: _____ _____

e. Awareness stage of adoption: _____ _____

f. Persuasion stage of adoption: _____ _____

g. Scientific merit: _____ _____

h. Cost/benefit assessment: _____ _____

2. Prepare an example of a research question that could be posed to improve nursing care in the five phases of the nursing process.

a. Assessment phase: _____ _____

 b. Diagnosis phase:

_____

_____

 c. Planning phase:

_____

_____

 d. Intervention phase:

_____

_____

 e. Evaluation phase:

_____

_____

3. Think about a nursing procedure about which you have been instructed. What is the basis for this procedure? Determine whether the procedure is based on scientific evidence that the procedure is effective. If it is not based on scientific evidence, on what is it based, and why do you think scientific evidence was not used?

4. Identify the factors in your own setting that you think facilitate or inhibit research utilization (or, in an education setting, the factors that promote or inhibit a climate in which research utilization is valued).

5. Read either Brett's (1987) article regarding the adoption of 14 nursing innovations ("Use of nursing practice research findings," *Nursing Research, 36,* 344–349), or the more recent study based on the same 14 innovations by Coyle and Sokop (1990) ("Innovation adoption behavior among nurses," *Nursing Research, 39,* 176–180). For each of the 14 innovations, indicate whether you: are aware of the findings; are persuaded that the findings should be used; use the findings sometimes in a clinical situation; or use the findings always in a clinical situation.

 1. _____

 2. _____

 3. _____

4. _____
5. _____
6. _____
7. _____
8. _____
9. _____
10. _____
11. _____
12. _____
13. _____
14. _____

6. With regard to the 14 innovations in Brett's study (see Question C.5 above), select an innovation or finding of which you (or most class members) were not aware. Go to the original source and read the research report. Perform a critique of the study, indicating in particular why you think there may have been barriers to having the innovation implemented in a local setting.

◩ D. APPLICATION EXERCISES

Below are several suggested research articles. Read one or more of these articles, paying special attention to the discussion and implications sections of the report. Evaluate the extent to which the researcher(s) facilitated the utilization of the study findings within clinical settings. If possible, suggest some clinical implications that the researchers did not discuss, or discuss the implications in terms of nursing education.

- Beach, E. K., Smith, A., Luthringer, L., Utz, S. K., Ahtens, S., & Whitmire, V. (1996). Self-care limitations of persons after acute myocardial infarction. (1996). *Applied Nursing Research, 9*, 24–28.
- Elliott, M. R., Drummond, J., & Barnard, K. E. (1996). Subjective appraisal of infant crying. *Clinical Nursing Research, 5*, 237–250.
- Failla, S., Kuper, B. C., Nick, T. G., & Lee, F. A. (1996). Adjustment of women with systemic lupus erythematosus. *Applied Nursing Research, 9*, 87–96.
- Rutman, D. (1996). Caregiving as women's work: Women's experiences of powerfulness and powerlessness as caregivers. *Qualitative Health Research, 6*, 90–111.
- Sandelowski, M., & Jones, L. C. (1996). Couples' evaluations of foreknowledge of fetal impairment, *Clinical Nursing Research, 5*, 81–96.

- Schilke, J. M., Johnson, G. O., Housh, T. J., & O'Dell, J. R. (1996). Effects of muscle-strength training on the functional status of patients with osteoarthritis of the knee joint. *Nursing Research, 45,* 68–72.

▨ E. SPECIAL PROJECTS

1. Select a study from the nursing research literature. Using the utilization criteria indicated in Boxes 14-1 and 14-2 of the text, assess the potential for utilizing the study results in a clinical practice setting. If the study meets the major criteria for utilization, develop a utilization plan.

2. Read the reports on the utilization project conducted under the auspices of the Association of Women's Health, Obstetric, and Neonatal Nurses (AWHONN):

- Meier, P. P. (1994). Transition of the preterm infant to an open crib: Process of the project group. *Journal of Obstetric, Gynecologic, and Neonatal Nursing, 23,* 321–326.
- Medoff-Cooper, B. (1994). Transition of the preterm infant to an open crib. *Journal of Obstetric, Gynecologic, and Neonatal Nursing, 23,* 329–335.
- Gelhar, D.. K., Miserendino, C. A., O'Sullivan, P. L., & Vessey, J. A. (1994). Research from the research utilization project: Environmental temperatures. *Journal of Obstetric, Gynecologic, and Neonatal Nursing, 23,* 341–344.

Evaluate the efficacy of this utilization project.

Research Reports

PART VII

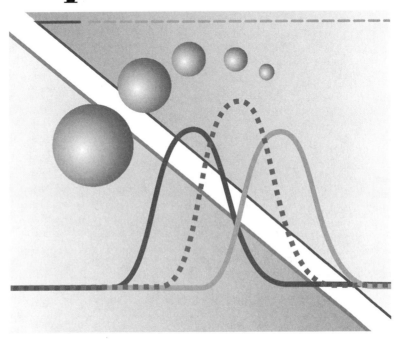

Effects of a Procedural/Belief Intervention on Breast Self-Examination Performance

Victoria Champion
Catherine Scott

The purpose of this study was to test the effect of a theoretically based nurse-delivered intervention on BSE behavior. A 2 × 2 prospective, randomized, factorial design yielded four groups: control, belief intervention, procedural intervention, and procedural/belief intervention. A total of 301 women were randomly selected from a target population. One year following intervention, significant differences in self-reported proficiency, observer-rated proficiency, and sensitivity (lump detection) were found between the Procedural and Control Group and the Procedural/Belief and Control Group. Significant increases were found on observer-rated proficiency and sensitivity for the Procedural/Belief Group when compared to the Belief Group. In addition, a significant increase was found in the Procedural/Belief Group on nodule detection, when compared to the Procedural Group alone. © 1993 John Wiley & Sons, Inc.

Victoria Champion, DNS, is a professor and Associate Dean for Research, School of Nursing, Indiana University. Catherine Scott, BSN, is a doctoral student in nursing at Indiana University.

This study was supported by NCNR Grant No. NR01843-03.

Champion, V., & Scott, C. (1993). Effects of a procedural/belief intervention on breast self-examination performance. *Research in Nursing and Health, 16,* 163–170. Reprinted with permission.

Requests for reprints can be addressed to Dr. Victoria Champion, Indiana University, School of Nursing, 1111 Middle Drive, Indianapolis, IN 46202-5107.

The incidence of breast cancer continues to rise. The most recent estimates indicate that 186,000 new breast cancers will be detected in the United States in 1992 (Boring, Squires, & Tong, 1992). The best way to lower mortality rates from breast cancer is early diagnosis; 91% of patients with breast cancer discovered at Stage I will be alive in 5 years as opposed to 18% of those whose tumors have advanced to Stage IV (American Cancer Society, 1991).

Breast self-examination (BSE) remains a recommended supplement to mammography and clinical breast examination for enhancing early detection of breast cancers. A number of investigators have found a mortality or stage benefit for women practicing BSE (Foster & Constanza, 1984; Huguley & Brown, 1981; Huguley, Brown, Greenberg, & Clark, 1988; Koroltchouck, Stanley & Stjernsward, 1990; Locker et al., 1989). The purpose of this study was to test selected belief and/or procedural interventions to increase self-reported BSE frequency and proficiency, observer-rated proficiency and sensitivity using a probability sample of women 35 years of age and older.

Many approaches have been used to examine the effects of interventions on increasing BSE frequency, proficiency and, in a few cases, sensitivity. Approaches have varied from handing out pamphlets to prospective randomized trials that include multiple interventions. Some investigators have measured only frequency as the outcome variable (Edgar & Shamian, 1987; Nettles-Carlson, Field, Friedman, & Smith, 1988); others have included proficiency and lump detection (Baines & To, 1990; Fletcher et al., 1990; Worden et al., 1990).

The Health Belief Model (HBM) has influenced research related to BSE behavior. According to the HBM, individuals who have a certain constellation of beliefs will be more likely to carry out a behavior (Rosenstock, 1966). Theoretically, beliefs associated with BSE would be perceived susceptibility to breast cancer, perceived seriousness of breast cancer, perceived benefits of BSE, and few perceived barriers to BSE. It follows, then, that interventions could be aimed at developing the optimal set of beliefs set forth by the HBM that would result in increased BSE behavior.

Health Belief Model (HBM) variables of perceived susceptibility to and seriousness of breast cancer, as well as perceived benefits of and barriers to BSE, have been related to BSE behavior (Champion, 1990; Lashley, 1987; Ronis & Kaiser, 1989; Rutledge, 1987). Worden, Constanza, Foster, Lang, and Tidd (1983) addressed beliefs about susceptibility and benefits using slide/tape presentations with women's groups. Six months after intervention BSE frequency had increased from 40 to 71%. Several other investigators have tested strategies aimed at changing beliefs to be theoretically consistent with the desired behavior (Baker, 1989; Calnan & Rutter, 1986; Carter, Feldman, Tierfer, & Hausdorff, 1985; Mahloch et al., 1990; Nettles-Carlson et al., 1988; Paskett et al., 1990; Worden et al., 1990). Baker (1989) found that a teaching strategy that included work with the HBM variables of susceptibility, seriousness, benefits, and barriers resulted in increased frequency and proficiency in a group of 194 older women 3 months after the intervention. Worden et al., (1990) found on a second year follow-up that women who had barriers addressed had higher scores for sensitivity, frequency, and proficiency than women who had not had this intervention.

Although there have been attempts to incorporate HBM variables into BSE interventions, more work is needed. Many investigators have used only frequency as an outcome measure without adequate attention to proficiency. Even when proficiency was considered, self-reported proficiency, with its potential for social desirability bias, was the primary measurement modality. In addition, short time intervals of 3 to 6 months without measures of long-term change often have been used. Finally, past approaches have not individualized teaching by evaluating pretest scores and addressing only salient belief variables. It is necessary to determine if individualized interventions to alter beliefs added to routine BSE teaching will increase BSE outcome behaviors over and above normal procedural teaching alone. Finally, we need valid and reliable measures of BSE, including observed proficiency and a measure of sensitivity (lump detection).

The 2×2 factorial design used for this study incorporated four groups: (a) control, (b) belief intervention, (c) procedural intervention and, (d) procedural/belief interventions. The HBM variables of perceived susceptibility, seriousness, benefits, barriers, health motivation, and control framed the belief intervention. The procedural intervention consisted of a standardized BSE teaching protocol, *Special Touch,* utilized by the American Cancer Society (American Cancer Society, 1987) that involved return demonstration and feedback. Observed proficiency and a measure of sensitivity (lump detection) were added to the measurements of outcome variables.

Hypotheses

1. There will be significant differences between experimental and control groups in self-reported frequency and proficiency of BSE and in observer-rated proficiency and sensitivity one year following intervention.
2. There will be significant increases in self-reported BSE frequency and proficiency and in observer-rated proficiency and sensitivity one year following intervention in the group receiving both belief and procedural protocols when compared to the groups receiving only one of these interventions.

▧ METHOD

Sample

Random-digit dialing was used to produce a probability sample of women 35 years and older who had not developed breast cancer. Telephone solicitors dialed computer-generated random numbers from a large midwestern metropolitan area and its surrounding counties. If there was not an answer, the number was redialed at least 10 times. When an eligible woman was contacted, the study was explained and the woman asked to participate. Women were randomly assigned to one of four groups and assessed on belief variables. An in-home interview was then conducted at which time the intervention was delivered. Women were interviewed one year following intervention to measure outcome variables.

Thirty-three percent of eligible women who were contacted agreed to participate in a larger longitudinal study ($2^1/_2$ years) and completed a baseline survey. Of the initial 322 women who completed the first two phases of data collection, 94% were available for follow-up one year later ($N = 301$).

Demographic characteristics of the sample population were similar to the general target population. Approximately 90% were white, 8% were black, and the remaining Asian or Indian. The mean age for the sample was 50 years ($SD = 12.15$), with a range from 35 to 88. The mean educational level was 13.7 years ($SD = 2.66$) with a range from 8 to 20. Women were paid $25.00 for each in-home interview.

Intervention

Belief Intervention. Women in the Belief and Procedural/Belief Groups who had belief scores at the midpoint or below for susceptibility, seriousness, benefits, and health motivation or control and midpoint or above for barriers were targeted for interventions. Belief interventions consisted of counseling individuals about their beliefs when they were not theoretically consistent with desired behavior. Pamphlets with appropriate belief messages were used in the intervention and left with the participant. For the susceptibility intervention, a pamphlet was used which described susceptibility factors for breast cancer. The individual's risk factors were also discussed. The seriousness pamphlet included statistics related to death from breast cancer. The benefits intervention explained the benefits of finding a lump early. The barriers pamphlet discussed common barriers women perceive in relation to BSE and offered suggestions to overcome these barriers. Health motivation and control interventions were aimed at increasing each woman's perception of the importance of general health and her personal control over health.

Extensive training and written materials were provided for research assistants. A training film was produced in which role modeling for each intervention was illustrated. In addition, the principal investigator trained the research assistants by watching them demonstrate the intervention and providing corrective feedback.

Procedural Intervention. A teaching program based on American Cancer Society recommendations for BSE procedure(s) was delivered to women in the Procedural and Procedural/Belief Groups (American Cancer Society, 1987). Registered nurse graduate students were trained and certified by the ACS to deliver the intervention. A breast model (Health Edco, 1992) was used for demonstrating BSE technique and for the return demonstration. Women were instructed to use adequate pressure for lump detection. Lumps were embedded in the model to allow women the experience of feeling a lump.

Measures

Measurement of HBM variables was accomplished by asking subjects to respond to a series of belief statements, with responses on summated 5-point Likert scales from *strongly agree* to *strongly disagree.* The scale included items for susceptibility, seriousness, benefits, barriers, health motivation, and control. The scales were originally developed by Champion (Champion, 1984) and revised extensively for this research project (Champion, in press). A panel of three national experts who had previously worked with the HBM theory assessed each item for content validity. Consensus was obtained before the item was retained.

All belief scales were assessed for criterion and construct validity. Construct validity was assessed by exploratory factor analysis. Criterion validity was assessed by correlating the entire scale and subscales (susceptibility, seriousness, benefits, barriers, health motivation, and control) with the criterion measure of BSE behavior ($R^2 = .24$, $p \leq .001$). Scales were tested for internal consistency and test-retest reliabilities. Internal consistency reliabilities were good and ranged from .80 to .93. Test-retest correlations were moderate, ranging from .45 to .70 (see Table 1). A time lag of between 2 to 8 weeks may have decreased test-retest reliabilities. In addition, the problem of testing effects may have lowered reliabilities, a problem addressed by Carmines and Zeller (1979). Extensive validity and reliability analyses were completed and are reported in detail elsewhere (Champion, in press).

Frequency and Proficiency of Self-Reports. Women were asked about the total number of times they had done BSE in the last 12 months (frequency) and about their technique (proficiency) using BSE behavior scales. Items assessed positioning of hands, areas of breasts covered, and other proficiency issues addressed by the American Cancer Society (American Cancer Society, 1987). All items were scored so that increasing magnitude indicated better practice. The BSE behavior scale had a Cronbach alpha of .73 and test-retest reliability of .74. Content validity

Table 1. Statistics for HBM Scales

Scale	M	SD	Cronbach Alpha	Test-Restest Correlation	# Items
Susceptibility	2.54	.81	.93	.70	6
Seriousness	3.25	.68	.80	.45	8
Benefits	3.88	.52	.80	.45	6
Barriers	2.02	.60	.88	.65	7
Health motivation	3.78	.59	.83	.67	8
Control	4.04	.55	.80	.46	4

was assessed by consensus of three experts who were BSE trainers. Confirmatory factor analyses established construct validity.

Observation of Proficiency. Participants were observed doing BSE on a model and their performance scored by the graduate nurse research assistant. Because some women were not comfortable returning a demonstration on themselves, all women were tested using the model. The observer checklist contained 10 procedural components that are important for BSE and that corresponded to items included in the self-report BSE measurement scale. Items included positioning of hands and breast area covered, as well as the other items listed in the self-report instrument. Participants were given 2 points for each of eight steps that were adequately completed. Participants were given 4 points each for the last two items since these items involved both position and examination of each breast. Partial credit was given when a step was only partially completed. A total of 24 points was possible on the proficiency checklist. An interobserver reliability of .90 was obtained by having four research assistants simultaneously score four different BSE demonstrations and calculating a coefficient based on the ratio of agreements to agreement plus disagreement.

Sensitivity. Participants were assessed on how many nodules embedded in a breast model (Health Edco, 1992) they could identify. A total of five nodules were embedded, and 1 point was given for each nodule identified.

Procedure

After being contacted by telephone and agreeing to participate, all subjects were sent the consent form and the initial survey to assess belief variables. The forms were completed and returned by mail (Time 1), after which research assistants scheduled in-home interviews (Time 2). A second in-home interview was conducted one year later (Time 3).

Subjects were randomly assigned to one of four groups prior to the in-home interview. For subjects assigned to Belief and Procedural/Belief Groups, research assistants used the initial survey to assess participants' scores on susceptibility, seriousness, benefits, barriers, health motivation, and control and to plan interventions when beliefs on any of the HBM variables were not consistent with desirable BSE behavior. Since BSE behavior is not considered adequate in the population generally, it was decided that an average or below average score on belief variables was not adequate to stimulate behavior; therefore, individuals who scored at or below the mean were targeted for intervention. In a like manner, barrier scores at or above the mean were addressed.

If a participant in the Belief Group did not need any of the belief interventions, only the data collection interview occurred at the first in-home visit. The Procedure-Only Group received the BSE teaching intervention as recommended by the ACS. If the participant was in the Procedural/Belief Group and did not require any belief intervention, the procedural intervention alone and data collection interview were conducted. The Control Group had an in-home interview in which all variables were again assessed but no intervention delivered. All groups had variables assessed a second time, with all but the Control Group having the assessment interview after the intervention was delivered. The time between Time 1 and Time 2 ranged from 2 to 8 weeks with a mean of about 4 weeks. One year following the initial in-home interview (Time 2), a second in-home interview (Time 3) was conducted for all groups to assess the effect of interventions on outcome variables.

All statistical analyses were done using SPSSx (Nie, 1988). *T* tests were used to test for significant differences between pre- and postintervention beliefs. A priori contrasts with a one-way ANOVA were used to test for differences in outcome measures between groups on measures that were collected only at Time 3. Self-reported BSE frequency and proficiency before and after interventions were assessed with MANOVA for repeated measures using Time 1 data as a covariate. The repeated measures program allows for testing of equality between groups at pretest and uses any variation (even if not significant) in analysis of posttest differences; it also allows for assessment of pre- to posttest differences across groups. In addition, the repeated measures analysis is more robust than a covariance approach, making it a preferable technique.

▧ RESULTS

A total of 147 participants from the Belief and the Procedural/Belief Group were given a belief intervention on at least one HBM variable. The numbers of subjects receiving each intervention were as follows: susceptibility (133), seriousness (135), benefits (111), barriers (125), health motivation (139), and control (106).

Baseline and postintervention measurement for all dependent measures are shown in Table 2. Groups were not significantly different on beliefs prior to intervention. Prior to hypotheses testing, data from the Belief and Procedural/Belief Groups were examined by correlated *t* tests (repeated measures) to determine if significant differences in beliefs emerged between pretest (Time 1) and immediately following intervention (Time 2). Belief and Procedural/Belief Groups were included in analysis since these were the only groups that had interventions aimed at changing beliefs. Significant differences in the expected direction emerged for all belief variables except susceptibility: seriousness $t = 6.25$, $p \le .001$; benefits $t = 7.50$, $p \le .001$; barriers $t = 4.02$, $p \le .001$; health motivation $t = 5.85$, $p \le .001$; and control $t = 4.43$, $p \le .001$).

An ANOVA indicated no significant differences between Experimental and Control in either frequency or proficiency prior to intervention. Hypothesis 1 predicted significant effects of intervention on self-reported frequency and proficiency, and observer rated proficiency and sensitivity. A repeated measures MANOVA (group × time) was used to test for intervention effects across time. A significant interaction effect between time and group was needed to indicate a true

Table 2. Pre/Postintervention Statistics for BSE Measures

	Control Group (N = 78)		Belief Group (N = 74)		Procedural Group (N = 75)		Procedural/ Belief Group (N = 73)	
	M	SD	M	SD	M	SD	M	SD
Frequency								
Preintervention	5.40	4.45	5.77	4.38	6.43	4.71	7.16	4.83
Postintervention[a]	9.44	4.05	10.54	3.35	10.40	3.10	11.00	2.51
Proficiency								
Preintervention	23.21	5.16	22.44	5.50	22.80	5.32	23.69	5.36
Postintervention[a]	28.23	5.21	28.15	5.84	31.21	4.34	31.77	4.00
Observation[a]	11.21	5.19	12.18	5.46	17.15	5.32	17.14	5.36
Nodules[a]	2.46	1.27	2.34	1.09	3.37	1.05	3.80	1.00

[a]Data collected 1 year postintervention.

intervention effect. Results indicated a significant increase in frequency across time $F(1,296) = 262.10$, $p \leq .001$. The group effect was also significant $F(3,296) = 3.23$, $p = .023$. The interaction effect, however, was nonsignificant, indicating that group differences at 1 year postintervention were due to the additive effect of pretest and posttest differences.

Self-reported proficiency data also were assessed using MANOVA with repeated measures. There was a significant difference in self-reported proficiency between groups $F(3,274) = 5.03$, $p \leq .002$, and across time, $F(1,274) = 281.62$, $p \leq .001$; the interaction effect also was significant, $F(3,274) = 5.69$, $p \leq .001$. The Procedural Only and Procedural/Belief Group had a greater increase in proficiency over time than those who received an intervention aimed at beliefs alone or no intervention. Planned comparisons indicated the Procedural and Procedural/Belief Groups, but not the Belief Group, were significantly different than the Control Group. Planned comparisons also indicated the Procedural and Procedural/Belief Groups were not significantly different in terms of proficiency.

Hypothesis 1 also stated that there would be a significant difference in observer-rated scores for proficiency and sensitivity between Experimental and Control Groups. Using a priori contrasts, the Control Group demonstrated significantly lower observer-rated proficiency and sensitivity than either the Procedural or the Procedural/Belief Group, but not the Belief Group (see Table 3).

To test hypothesis 2, behavioral outcomes of the Procedural/Belief intervention were compared to those of the Belief and Procedural interventions. A priori contrasts between the Belief and Procedural/Belief Group were significant for both the observer-

Table 3. A Priori Contrasts for Observer-Rated Proficiency and Sensitivity

	Observer Rated Proficiency *t* Value (*df* = 294)	Sensitivity *t* Value (*df* = 295)
Control versus belief	1.02	.68
Control versus procedural	6.24*	5.03*
Control versus procedural/belief	6.18*	7.40*
Procedural versus procedural/belief	.02	2.35*
Belief versus procedural/belief	5.10*	7.98*

*$p \leq .01$.

rated proficiency and sensitivity scores, with the Procedural/Belief Group attaining higher proficiency (see Table 3). A priori contrasts between the Procedural Group and Procedural/Belief Group intervention revealed significant differences for sensitivity (see Table 3). The mean sensitivity for the Procedural Group was 3.36 (*SD* = 1.05) as compared to 3.80 (*SD* = .99) for the Procedural/Belief Group. A limited range (5 lumps) may have precluded finding greater differences.

◩ DISCUSSION

Self-reported retrospective frequency scores for BSE were not significantly different between groups when pretest differences were controlled. There were significant increases in frequency between pre- and postintervention scores, however, even in the Control Group. This finding probably indicates that the effect of being in the study sensitized women to report increased BSE frequency. Individual attention did act to increase reported frequency and this increase was maintained for 1 year. This result may be important considering that maintaining behavior over time has been found to be difficult (Mayer et al., 1987).

Self-reported proficiency scores illustrate a different pattern. Scores for the Procedural and Procedural/Belief Groups increased more over time than scores for the Control or Belief Groups, indicating an effect from the Procedural and Procedural/Belief interventions. It is also obvious that since frequency differences between groups were nonsignificant when proficiency differences were significant, that frequency alone is not an adequate measure of BSE behavior, thus calling into question reports of studies that address only frequency (Edgar & Shamian, 1987; Nettles-Carlson et al., 1988).

Demonstrations of BSE on models were not done on pretest to partially control for the sensitizing effect of demonstrating the procedure. In addition, since this was a randomized design, groups could be assumed equal on these measures. Nurse-rated proficiency 1 year after intervention was higher in the groups that had received training in the procedure, confirming the usefulness of that intervention. Observer-rated proficiency is probably a more valid indicator of actual technique than are self-report measures since it avoids the problem of self-report bias.

The most important findings are the significant differences that emerged in terms of sensitivity. Both the Procedural Group and the Procedural/Belief Groups were significantly different from the Control or Belief Groups. In addition, the Procedural/Belief Group was significantly different than the group receiving only procedural instruction. Having a theoretically consistent set of beliefs may increase the desire for learning which results in the procedural intervention being more effective. This finding is especially important in light of the need for research with better outcome measures (O'Malley & Fletcher, 1987). This finding also is consistent with Worden et al. (1990), who found that a group in which barriers were assessed had increased sensitivity (lump detection). The possibility must be acknowledged, however, that detection of lumps in a synthetic model would not translate to actual lump detection. It also is difficult to assess the clinical significance of this finding. In addition, false-positive lump identification was not measured in this study. It would be impossible, however, to design a study using lump detection in a human as the outcome measure without conducting an extremely large longitudinal study that would extend for years. This study did incorporate the most logical analogue to lump detection in women (lump detection in a synthetic model) an improvement over other studies (Baker, 1989; Grady, 1988; Nettles-Carlson, et al., 1988).

Because this study took place in the participant's home, the results cannot be generalized to clinic settings. There is no reason to think, however, that results would be different in a clinic, and it is even possible that individualized interventions would be more effective when delivered in a medical or health care setting. Although group differences in postintervention self-reported frequency were not found, frequency increases over time were significant for all groups. The effect of intervention with a nurse may have acted as an intervention even for the Control Group. Further research with a no-cantact control group may help clarify this finding.

It is encouraging that a high percentage of women (94%) remained in the study after initial intervention. The somewhat low proportion of subjects who initially agreed to participate (33%) does limit generalization. However, refusal to participate was often attributed to reluctance to commit to a $2^{1}/_{2}$ year study and, therefore, it is not surprising that the refusal rate for this study was higher than the rates for cross-sectional studies. It also must be acknowledged that, although approximately 95% of women in the target population had a telephone, results cannot be generalized to those without phones. Generalizability is also limited because participants were relatively well educated and may have been more interested in or motivated to learn about BSE than those who refused. This limitation, however, is common in research with volunteer subjects.

In conclusion, preliminary results indicate that nursing interventions may increase BSE frequency and proficiency over time. Personal contact emphasizing

BSE may be all that is needed to increase frequency; however, proficiency was dependent upon a standardized teaching Procedure and/or Procedural/Belief intervention. The lack of difference between Procedural and Procedural/Belief Groups on some outcome measures may have been due in part to the fact that the teaching intervention (the American Cancer Society protocol) also included emphasis on decreasing barriers and increasing control over health, as well as information about susceptibility. Follow-up over longer periods is needed to provide information on long-term effects.

These preliminary findings indicate a statistically significant additive effect for sensitivity when belief interventions are added to procedural teaching. If this is confirmed in subsequent studies, the cost effectiveness of this additional step in teaching BSE should be examined. In addition, targeted and individualized interventions should be compared to a standardized format in which all women receive the same belief intervention regardless of individualized differences.

▧ REFERENCES

American Cancer Society. (1987). *Speech touch facilitators guide,* Atlanta: Author.

American Cancer Society. (1991). *Cancer facts & figures—1991,* Atlanta: Author.

Baines, C. J., & To, T. (1990). Changes in breast self-examination behavior achieved by 89,835 participants in the Canadian National Breast Screening Study. *Cancer, 66,* 570–576.

Baker, J. A. (1989). Breast self-examination and the older woman: Field testing an educational approach. *The Gerontologist,* 29, 405–407.

Boring, M. S., Squires, T., & Tong, T. (1991). Cancer statistics, 1992. *CA—A Cancer Journal for Clinicians, 42*(1), 19–38.

Calnan, M., & Rutter, D. R. (1986). Do health beliefs predict health behaviour? An analysis of breast self-examination. *Social Science & Medicine, 22,* 673–678.

Carmines, E., & Zeller, P. (1979). *Reliability and validity assessment.* Newbury Park, CA: Sage.

Carter, A. C., Feldman, J. G., Tierfer, L., & Hausdorff, J. K. (1985). Methods of motivating the practice of breast self-examination: A randomized trial. *Preventive Medicine, 14,* 555–572.

Champion, V. L. (1984). Instrument development for health belief model constructs. *Advances in Nursing, Science, 6*(3), 73–85.

Champion, V. L. (1990). Breast self-examination in women 35 and older: A prospective study. *Journal of Behavioral Medicine, 13,* 523–528.

Champion, V. L. (in press). Refinement of instruments to measure Health Belief Model constructs. *Nursing Research.*

Edgar, L., & Shamian, J. (1987). Promoting healthy behaviours: The nurse as a teacher of breast self-estamination. *HYGIE, 6*(2), 37–41.

Fletcher, S. W., O'Malley, M. S., Earp, J. A. L., Morgan, T. M., Lin, S., & Degnan, D. (1990). How best to teach women breast self-examination. A randomized controlled trial. *Annals of Internal Medicine, 112,* 772–779.

Foster, R. S., & Constanza, M. C. (1984). Breast self-examination practices and breast cancer survival. *Cancer, 53,* 999–1005.

Grady, K. E. (1988). Older women and the practice of breast self-examination. *Psychology of Women Quarterly, 12,* 473–487.

Health Edco. (1992). *Educational products catalog.* Waco, TX.

Huguley, C. M., & Brown, R. L. (1981). The value of breast self-examination. *Cancer, 47,* 989–995.

Huguley, C., Brown, R., Greenberg, R., & Clark, S. (1988). Breast self-examination and survival from breast cancer. *Cancer, 62,* 1389–1396.

Koroltchouk, V., Stanley, K., & Stjernsward, J. (1990). The control of breast cancer. A World Health Organization perspective. *Cancer, 65,* 2803–2810.

Lashley, M. E. (1987). Predictors of breast self-examination practice among elderly women. *Advances in Nursing Science, 9*(4), 25–34.

Locker, A., Caseldine, J., Mitchell, A., Blamey, R., Roebuck, E., & Elston, C. (1989). Results from a seven-year programme of breast self-examination in 89,010 women. *British Journal of Cancer, 60,* 401–405.

Mahloch, J., Paskett, E., Henderson, M., Grizzle, J., Ross-Price, M., & Thompson, R. S. (1990). An evaluation of BSE frequency and quality and their relationship to breast lump detection. *Progress in Clinical & Biological Research, 339,* 269–280.

Mayer, J. A., Dubbert, P. M., Scott, R. R., Dawson, B. L., Ekstrand, M. L., & Fondren, T. G. (1987). Breast self-examination: The effects of personalized prompts on practice frequency. *Behavior Therapy, 2,* 135–146.

Nettles-Carlson, B., Field, M. L., Friedman, B. J., & Smith, L. S. (1988). Effectiveness of teaching breast self-examination during office visits. *Research in Nursing & Health, 11,* 41–50.

Nie, N. H. (1988). *SPSSx user's guide.* New York: McGraw-Hill.

O'Malley, M. S., & Fletcher, S. W. (1987). Screening for breast cancer with breast self-examination. *Journal of the American Medical Association, 257,* 2197–2203.

Paskett, E. D., White, E., Urban, N., Gey, G. O., Hornecker, J., Meadows, S., & Sifferman, F. R. (1990). Implementation and evaluation of a worksite breast self-examination training program. *Progress in Clinical & Biological Research, 339,* 281–302.

Ronis, D. L., & Kaiser, M. K. (1989). Correlates of breast self-examination in a sample of college women: Analyses of linear structural relations. *Journal of Applied Social Psychology, 19,* 1068–1084.

Rosenstock, I. M. (1966). Why people use health services. *Milbank Memorial Fund Quarterly, 44,* 94–121.

Rutledge, D. M. (1987). Factors related to women's practice of breast self-examination. *Nursing Research, 36,* 117–121.

Worden, J. K., Constanza, M. C., Foster, R. S., Lang, S. P., & Tidd, C. A. (1983). Content and context in health education: Persuading women to perform breast self-examination. *Preventive Medicine, 12,* 331–339.

Worden, J. K., Solomon, L. J., Flynn, B. S., Constanza, M. C., Foster, R. S., Dorwaldt, A. L., & Weaver, S. O. (1990). A community-wide program in breast self-examination training and maintenance. *Preventive Medicine, 19,* 254–269.

AIDS Family Caregiving: Transitions Through Uncertainty*

Marie Annette Brown
and Gail M. Powell-Cope†

The purpose of this study was to describe the experience of AIDS family caregiving. Grounded theory provided the methodological basis for qualitative data generation and analysis. Extensive interviews were conducted with 53 individuals (lovers, spouses, parents of either adults or children with AIDS, siblings, and friends) who were taking care of a person with AIDS at home. Relevant features of the social context of AIDS family caregiving were explored. Findings revealed the basic social psychological problem of Uncertainty, a core category of Transitions Through Uncertainty, and five subcategories: Managing and Being Managed by the Illness; Living With Loss and Dying; Renegotiating the Relationship; Going Public; and Containing the Spread of HIV. Stages and strategies of each subcategory detailed individuals' responses to the challenges of AIDS family caregiving and elaborated the day-to-day experiences. Uncertainty as a critical challenge for individuals and families facing life-threatening illness is discussed in light of recent research.

*Accepted for publication April 8, 1991. Earlier versions of this paper were presented at the 1989 meeting of the Western Institute for Nursing and the 1989 Council of Nurse Researchers meeting. This study was funded in part by a Biomedical Research Support Grant from the University of Washington School of Nursing and the Psi Chapter of Sigma Theta Tau. Although there is a designated first and second author, this article is a result of a collaborative effort between the authors. Both authors contributed equally to the final product. We gratefully acknowledge the generous contribution of time from our study participants. We sincerely appreciate the substantive and methodological assistance provided by Kristen Swanson, PhD, RN, Phil Bereano, PhD, Kimberly Moody, PhC, RN, and Linda Meldman, PhC, RN.

Reprinted here from *Nursing Research* (1991; 40[6]:338–345), with permission.

†Marie Annette Brown, PhD, RN, is an associate professor in the School of Nursing, University of Washington, Seattle, WA.

Gail M. Powell-Cope, PhC, RN, is a doctoral candidate in nursing science at the school of Nursing, University of Washington, Seattle, WA.

The physical and emotional devastation of HIV infection and AIDS produces extraordinary challenges to the health care system. Families and significant others assume heavy responsibilities for care of these individuals and provide the cornerstone of society's response to the AIDS epidemic (Haque, 1989; Wolcott et al., 1986). For example, Raveis and Siegel (1990) found that informal or familial caregivers provided approximately two-thirds of the total assistance required for instrumental activities, transportation, administrative activities, and home medical care for persons with AIDS (PWAs) even though the sample was relatively healthy. Hepburn (1990) emphasized that if family caregivers of PWAs "play a comparable role to informal caregivers of the elderly, they will have significant impact on the overall care and well-being of AIDS patients" (p. 41).

▧ LITERATURE REVIEW

The literature suggests that there are risks to assuming the family caregiver role of an elderly or ill person including physical morbidity (Snyder & Keefe, 1985; Baumgarten, 1989); depression, mental exhaustion, and burnout (Chenoweth & Spencer, 1986; Ekberg, Griffith, & Foxall, 1986; Livingston, 1985); burden, strain (Montgomery, Gonyea, & Hooyman, 1985; Zarit, Todd, & Zarit, 1986); anger, depression, and fatigue (Rabins, Mace, & Lucas, 1982; Rabins, Fitting, Eastham, & Fettig, 1990); and uncertainty (Stetz, 1989). Furthermore, parent caregivers of chronically ill children experience changes in the marital relationship, financial constraints, and role alterations (Thomas, 1987). These parent caregivers often become socially isolated as they focus on the ill child, become less available for reciprocal exchange with others, and experience the withdrawal of friends and other family members (Thomas, 1987). It is particularly common that middle-aged caregivers are unable to fulfill their work and family roles adequately (Miller & Montgomery, 1990). In a recent study of informal caregivers of PWAs, alterations in work role performance and economic burden were common, even though the sample consisted of relatively healthy PWAs with few functional disabilities (Raveis & Siegel, 1990). Over one-third of the caregivers had made financial changes in their lives and passed up financial opportunities, and 13% reported somewhat serious financial problems. Most (72%) of those employed reported that their ability to concentrate at work was affected by the patient's illness. A substantial minority (39%) reported arriving at work late or leaving early because the PWA was ill, had to be escorted to a medical appointment, or needed assistance with errands. Twenty-eight percent admitted that in recent months they had to take sick leave, vacation, or personal days because of the PWA's illness (Raveis & Siegel, 1990).

While there may be challenges common for all caregivers, each subgroup of caregivers faces unique psychosocial stressors, often related to the characteristics of the care recipient. Issues of communicability, stigma, and multiple and premature losses are common in AIDS family caregiving. The issue of communicability of this "deadly disease" can stimulate fears of contagion and death in loved ones, friends, and coworkers of both the patient and the family caregiver (Ostrow & Gayle, 1986). Coping with AIDS phobia, the stigma associated with homosexuality, bisexuality, or IV drug use, as well as the tremendous demands of caregiving, may become overwhelming for family members (Moffatt, 1986). Schoen (1986) highlighted the additional strain faced by younger caregivers, particularly spouses and lovers, who deal with such a catastrophic, life-threatening illness before reaching half of their life expectancy, and who have not acquired the maturity and perspective that often accompany middle and older age. Caregivers who are HIV positive witness deterioration and death that could forecast their own fate (Shilts, 1987; Edwards, 1988). Lastly, a large proportion of AIDS family caregivers are men, who in American culture usually receive less preparation than women for nurturing roles.

Virtually no information exists about AIDS family caregiving, and much of the general family caregiving research focuses only on caregiving tasks and related effects on the caregiver (Bowers, 1987). The grounded theory method is a particularly important research strategy to address these gaps and serves to "clarify, develop, or redirect research in a content area about which much is already known" (Bowers, 1987, p. 31). Therefore, the purpose of this grounded theory study was to explore and describe the experience of family members who were caring for PWAs at home. The term *family caregiver* employed in this study includes family of origin and family of choice.

▧ METHOD

Sample

Participants were recruited from a variety of AIDS community sources, including clinics, support groups, a caregiver course, volunteer organizations, and a community newspaper. The sample consisted of 53 family caregivers of people with symptomatic HIV infection or AIDS. Approximately one-third (32%) were partners or lovers in gay relationships, 6% were partners or spouses in heterosexual relationships, 43% were friends (9% were former lovers), 13% were parents, 4% were siblings, and 4% were other family of origin. The parents included those of both adult and minor children with HIV/AIDS. Seventy-seven percent lived in the same household with the PWA and 60% of the households also included other individuals such as the caregiver's partner, child, or housemate. Approximately two-thirds (64%) of the family caregivers were male and 36% were female. Approximately two-thirds (68%) were gay or bisexual and 32% were heterosexual. The sample ranged from 22 to 65 years old ($M = 36$). Fifty-seven percent had less than a college degree and 92% were white. Fifty percent of the caregivers were employed full-time and 19% part-time outside the home. Family incomes (which supported an average of 1.9 persons) were low, with 18% reporting under $10,000, 41% between $10–20,000, 16% $20–30,000, 16% $30–40,000, and 9% over $40,000. In almost half (47%) of the families, the PWA had been diagnosed within the past 12 months. Eighty-four percent of the caregivers knew the PWA prior to the diagnosis of AIDS. The sample contained few ethnic minorities and a large number of caregivers of gay PWAs, thus reflecting the demographics of AIDS in the geographical area where the study was conducted (DSHS & Seattle-King County Health Department, 1991). However, compared to family caregivers of people with other health problems, this sample was younger with a greater proportion of men, fewer spouses, and few members from families of origin.

Procedure

After consent was obtained, participants were asked: "What has it been like for you living with and taking care of someone with AIDS?" Relevant probes were used to gain further insight into issues raised. In addition, an interview guide was used to insure consistency of topics across interviews. Interviews were conducted in either one or two sessions, lasted a mean of 4.5 hours, and yielded over 200 hours of interview data. Confidentiality was maintained.

While a triangulation of methods was used to address the study purpose, this paper will include only findings from qualitative analyses. Grounded theory (Glaser & Strauss, 1967; Strauss, 1987) provided the methodological basis for qualitative data generation and analysis. This approach is derived from symbolic interactionism, which focuses on human social and psychological processes as they are grounded in social interaction. The basic tenet of symbolic interactionism is that people construct meanings about phenomenon based on interpretations of interactions they have with one another and with themselves (Blumer, 1969). Therefore, family caregiving is viewed as a socially interactive process that supports the ill person, in this case, the person with HIV infection.

Interviews were tape-recorded and transcribed verbatim. Constant comparative analysis was used as an ongoing technique that included deriving first level codes, or in vivo codes, comparing codes to one another, deriving conceptual categories, and relating categories to codes and to other categories. Coding strategies included open coding (unrestricted selection of codes from the search for words or phrases that capture the meaning in the transcripts), axial coding (comparison between codes), and selective coding (utilization of frequently occurring codes to create core categories). Theoretical sampling was accomplished by selecting respondents based on the need to collect more data to examine categories and their relationships, and to ensure representativeness in the category. Theoretical saturation determined the discontinuation of new data collection. Theoretical saturation occurred when information became redundant and a core category was created and linked to subcategories.

Validity and reliability of the data were addressed systematically using the criteria outlined by Sandelowski (1986) and Lincoln and Guba (1985): (a) truth value, (b) applicability, (c) consistency, and (d) neutrality. Member checks, debriefing by peers, triangulation, prolonged engagement with the data, persistent observation, and reflective journals were techniques used to ensure validity and reliability. During the final phases of analysis, focus groups of study alumni, family caregivers who did not participate in the study, and professionals and community volunteers working in the area of AIDS family caregiving were asked to review and to critique the validity of the substantive theory of AIDS family caregiving. Modifications of the theoretical presentation were made based on feedback from these experts as well as from consensus between the researchers. The categories developed during this study were also validated using literature in the popular press. Examination of Monette's (1988) detailed account of caring for his partner with AIDS revealed evidence of the basic social psychological problem, core category, subcategories, and stages and strategies.

Context and Assumptions

Grounded theory and methodology suggest that it is crucial to examine the broader social context of the phenomenon under study. The data from this study represent caregiving that occurred between 1985 and 1988. Caregiving during those years of the AIDS epidemic was inextricably linked to several salient issues: a silent government, a vocal gay community, an unresponsive bureaucracy, inexperienced health care providers, and a frightened, uninformed, and homophobic populace.

Specific aspects of the cultural context can be related to the five subcategories describing caregivers' responses to the challenge of AIDS. For example, complicating the caregivers' attempt to manage the illness was a society that undervalued care provided in the home and traditionally expected women to fulfill that role without compensation or reward. Living with loss and dying was made more difficult by the high value placed on youth and appearance. Pervasive divorce and domestic violence as well as widespread intolerance of nontraditional family compositions undermined the ability to maintain relationships. Because of the societal stigma associated with AIDS and fear of exposure to prejudice, persons with AIDS and caregivers were not encouraged to "go public" with their disease, but instead had to hide the truth.

Moreover, the attempt to contain the spread of HIV was hindered by contradictory messages. On one hand, popular images promoted by the media and embraced by society suggested that romantic sex should ideally be spontaneous and unprotected. While on the other hand, the medical community advised condom use to prevent the transmission of AIDS. Yet despite the information provided by the medical community, their efforts to convince the general public to practice "safe" sex were not adequate.

◪ **RESULTS**

The substantive theory of AIDS family caregiving developed during this study is outlined in Figure 1. *Uncertainty* was identified as the basic social psychological problem and *Transitions Through Uncertainty* the core category of AIDS family caregiving. In addition to the pervasive sense of uncertainty that characterized the

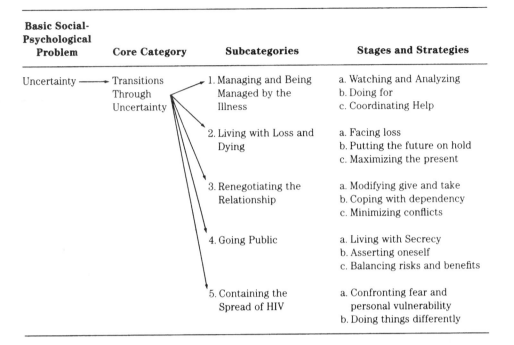

Figure 1. Substantive Theory of AIDS Family Caregiving

AIDS caregiving transition, the day-to-day experience of uncertainty was best understood in the context of the five caregiving subcategories (Figure 1). These subcategories provide a structure for detailing the multiple aspects of uncertainty. The subcategories also highlighted areas of caregivers' lives that were most significant and problematic. Stages and strategies of each subcategory detail caregivers' action-oriented responses to the uncertainties and specific challenges characteristic of each subcategory.

Uncertainty[1]

Uncertainty was identified as the basic social psychological problem in the AIDS caregiving transition. Uncertainty, as conceptualized in this study, is defined as the caregiver's inability to predict future events and outcomes and the lack of confidence in making day-to-day decisions about the ill person's care. Uncertainty exerted a profound influence on caregivers' lives and pervaded the entire caregiving experience; it never completely disappeared, but varied in intensity, timing, and

---

[1]Although our analysis was conducted without knowledge of Mishel's reconceptualization of the uncertainty in illness theory (1990), the studies contain parallel findings that support an expanded perspective on the acceptance of uncertainty.

content. Even though caregivers reported increasing confidence in their caregiving abilities and increasing ability to predict outcomes over time, uncertainty about some issue always remained. Even after one year of caregiving, one lover expressed some self-doubts.

> *So I don't necessarily feel 100% about everything I'm doing, but I have to do it . . . I'm not 100% positive, 100% sure, 100% that it's the right thing to do for Mike . . . It becomes very obscure, blurry, as to whether I'm doing anything right.*

Feelings of uncertainty in AIDS family caregiving arose from the perpetual and unpredictable changes accompanying AIDS. The PWA's health or functional ability and the caregivers' emotional responses were often in a constant state of flux. One caregiver emphasized the difficulties in trying to keep abreast of these constant changes:

> *It constantly changes. I want to emphasize that. You can't learn what the boundary is, because the boundary of today is not gonna be the boundary of tomorrow. What you've got to learn is how to have an antenna.*

Often, study participants spontaneously offered the roller coaster metaphor to describe the constant changes inherent in AIDS caregiving. A roller coaster, with many ups and downs, reflected the relentlessness and the lack of control in AIDS family caregiving. For the most part, caregivers were unable to seek respite from the constant drama of AIDS, and to create a more stable period in their lives. Two different caregivers expressed their feelings about the roller coaster as follows:

> *The roller coaster describes the situation in lots of different ways. What's happening to the person's health? What's happening to your feelings? What's happened here today? It's this incredible uncertainty.*

> *Well, it got to be like an emotional roller coaster, one of these up and down and up and down . . . So it's almost as though you want to tell yourself, well, his condition is stabilized. This stuff doesn't stabilize very long . . .*

Uncertainty was problematic for caregivers because of a cultural context that emphasizes the need to understand, predict, and/or control events. Caregivers struggled as they faced the contradiction between their expectations about prediction and control and the reality of their personal experiences which were imbued with constant uncertainty. Initially, caregivers expected health care providers to be able to provide them with incontestable information about AIDS and the PWA's course of illness. Caregivers often were frustrated when they turned to health care providers for definitive answers and found that the professionals were themselves equally uncertain. One caregiver expressed his frustration with the inability of the physicians to explain his partner's new and foreboding neurological symptoms:

> *He's got a malfunction in his brain and no one knows*
> *what's going on. The neurosurgeons, and neurologists and*
> *doctors at the AIDS clinic ... No one knows what's happening,*
> *but it's getting worse.*

While some caregivers learned to accept uncertainty over time, others had a stronger need to establish some degree of certainty in their lives. Some caregivers did not want to accept the uncertainty of AIDS caregiving and tried to force certainty where it did not exist. After numerous attempts to exercise control in the face of constant change, many caregivers discovered the fallacy of this imperative and began to accept uncertainty. One caregiver poignantly described his paradoxical reflections about the uncertainty of his lover's mortality:

> *I like to know what's going to happen in a clear-cut path*
> *in a pattern that I can control ... So my certainty was that I fi-*
> *nally decided Mike was going to die. Finally I realized what*
> *right do I have to decide the fate of someone else's life? He may*
> *not die. I was doing it for my own protection, my own sanity*
> *... So I opened up that wound, or whatever you call that, and*
> *let uncertainty back into my life.*

Transitions

A transition is a period of major change in life circumstances accompanied by uncertainty, questioning one's basic assumptions, and reexamining plans for living in the world (Parkes, 1971) which results in the reordering of life activities and a transformed self-identity. As a result of prolonged engagement with the data and with the literature, we identified caregiving as a transition to be a critical feature of AIDS family caregiving. Study participants consistently described AIDS caregiving as a significant phase of life as portrayed in the definition above. Many emphasized caregiving as a process that occurred over time or a series of changes. This lover struggled with the effects of dramatic changes in the PWA's health over a short period of time:

> *You should have talked to me three months ago when he*
> *was in the hospital with pneumonia. Life was completely dif-*
> *ferent then: I was a basket case, whirling from the news from*
> *AIDS and afraid of death at any moment. Now he's back to*
> *work and we seem to be pretending that we are living a nor-*
> *mal life.*

Others viewed caregiving as a journey or passage, or a path they chose. One man talked about his depth of experience as a caregiver for his lover:

> *If [caregiving] has been a real path ... It's a strange time*
> *for us right now. It's almost a very spiritual time.*

Caregiving may last for only a few months or extend over several years. As in any transition, caregiving demanded time for making meaning of events and experiences as caregivers learned to live and to view their worlds differently. Two partners described the common theme of a life transformed by AIDS caregiving:

> *Joe was diagnosed a little over one year ago and my life has changed forever . . . things keep happening . . . and I have discovered this past year how much work it is.*

> *He was diagnosed in May with a Kaposi's spot. Up until that time AIDS had never entered our relationship. Nobody ever thought about AIDS . . . It's completely changed our lives in a lot of ways. And where we're at right now is . . . we've almost come full circle now. We've worked out a lot of things this past year, dealing with the disease.*

The transition of AIDS caregiving was characterized by both numerous crises and quiescent periods between crises. Common precipitators of crises were usually associated with sudden changes in the PWA's health such as *Pneumocystis* pneumonia, falls, delirium, and acute panic attacks. One caregiver described his frightening experience of finding his lover at home critically ill:

> *I called him at his apartment and he was very, very sick and he was in a lot of denial. And the reality of it was that he was developing cryptococcal meningitis. He was becoming demented and totally out of it . . . He kept dropping the phone and not picking it up. I'd scream into the phone and there'd be no answer . . . finally I said, "I think we've got to go into the hospital." I went to pick him up and he had difficulty buzzing me into the apartment. When I got into the apartment it was a total mess. There was rotting food all over. He didn't know who he was.*

The quiescent times between crises were often viewed by caregivers as "good times." Often during these periods caregivers were able to focus more on their own lives, to create a more peaceful existence, and to increase involvement in community and social activities. One lover, who had experienced many crises with the PWA in the past year, now felt a respite from the difficulties and was enjoying a new sense of well-being.

> *It sounds hard to believe after all these things I've been telling you, but I'm very happy with the way my life is going right now. I have the most wonderful balance in the world, of working at the bakery part-time and being able to live in a very bohemian lifestyle, working in my garden, spending what time I can with Jeff. I am at definitely the most content place in my life than I've been in many, many, many years. I don't think I would do anything different right now.*

Managing and Being Managed by the Illness

This subcategory is defined as vigilantly monitoring the mercurial illness of HIV/AIDS and constantly responding to the relentless demands and uncertainties associated with caregiving tasks. The stages and strategies involved in *Managing and Being Managed* include (a) watching and analyzing, (b) doing for,[2] and (c) coordinating help.

Although present in all categories, uncertainty was most dramatic in *Managing and Being Managed* and reflected the recent appearance of AIDS as a new and poorly understood disease. This uncertainty for caregivers was related to questioning how the disease would unfold, monitoring the symptoms, determining the meaning of symptoms and illness behavior, deciding about treatment options, evaluating the effectiveness of caregiving strategies, and developing confidence in their ability to care for the PWA.

A common example of uncertainty related to monitoring the illness was the attempt to determine the meaning of the PWA's symptoms. This process was evident in the dilemma called, "Is it him or the disease?" Caregivers often questioned the PWA's behavior by asking, "Is this an emotional response to the disease (e.g., depression) or is this just him?" The uncertainty manifest in this question prompted caregivers to be cautious so that they would not overlook important symptoms. Consequently, they seriously questioned whether each symptom indicated a new manifestation of the disease, such as a brain lesion, the beginning of an opportunistic infection, or a milestone suggesting a slow, steady deterioration. In the absence of a physiological explanation, caregivers attempted to resolve the uncertainty by attributing symptoms to the PWA's personality. This form of uncertainty was often very stressful, as expressed by one woman caring for her friend:

> *His decision-making skills and abilities could be really impaired and it's important to keep a scope on that in your heads . . . It's like, he's crazy now! You know, it's hard to tell, because like I said, he's a pretty far out there person anyway. It's like, "Do you think he's crazy now? What do you guys think? I don't know . . . Maybe." . . . I mean, he goes out and buys a $300 funeral outfit. Is this crazy behavior?*

Being Managed by the Illness resulted from the relentless nature of caregiving activities and seriousness of the PWA's immune system compromised by HIV infection. Despite the numerous activities involved in managing the illness, the feeling of "never being able to do enough" contributed to the perception of being managed. One mother described how the vigilance of monitoring the disease and the uncertainty of the PWA's behavior translated into the feeling of "24 hours a day on call":

---

[2]The language and conceptualization of *Doing For* was influenced by Dr. Kristen Swanson's theoretical development of caring published in *Nursing Research* (Vol. 40, No. 3).

*You can't leave him alone too long because you never
know how the mind's going to be. You never know things. Like
one time I went to sleep and I thought he was in his room and
he had checked himself back into the hospital.*

For many caregivers, this constant vigilance became a major contributor to
the experience of *Being Managed by the Illness*. Overall, the cumulative stresses
associated with *Being Managed by the Illness* sometimes resulted in caregiver
burnout that seriously affected the individual's quality of life.

Living with Loss and Dying

This subcategory is defined as the process of revising one's plans for living in the
world based on the possible or probable death of a loved one. Stages and strategies
include: (a) Facing loss, (b) Putting the future on hold, and (c) Maximizing the
present.

Three major sources of uncertainty within *Living with Loss and Dying* were
described by caregivers: whether to remain hopeful about the PWA's survival, not
knowing which illness or opportunistic infection would herald the PWA's death, or
now knowing when the death would occur. These uncertainties related to facing
loss were very painful for caregivers to contemplate. Yet, death was so commonplace in those with AIDS, and the threat of death so powerful, that most caregivers
were unable to deny the reality of a probable death. One man described the uncertainty of his partner's survival during an acute illness:

*The doctor said, "You know I don't know . . ." Well, actu-
ally when Matt first went into the hospital he was so sick the
doctor said, "I don't know if he'll live through the evening or
he'll live for . . ." As the doctor told me, "He might die tonight,
he might die in six months," That was the time for him given.
And I thought, "Well, hmmm, this is an interesting situation."*

Another man wondered how the dying process of his lover would unfold:

*Sometimes I wonder "Will he, you know, will his im-
mune system just sort of fall apart, and will he have multiple
opportunists and die fairly quickly, within a matter of a few
months, or will there be a prolonged time of morbidity, lots of
time in the hospital, lots of time in which he feels bad and
needs emotional support from me and dies?"*

Both the long-range and short-term future were constant sources of uncertainty for caregivers. Even plans for the most immediate future—tomorrow, this
weekend—were always uncertain because they were contingent on the PWA's
strength and symptomology. Living "one day at a time" became an anchor in the
lives of many caregivers as they struggled with an uncertain future and focused on
the present.

Renegotiating the Relationship

This subcategory is defined as the ongoing process of revising the rules and expectations and striving to reach acceptable balances. Stages and strategies include (a) Modifying give and take, (b) Coping with dependency, and (c) Minimizing conflict. Uncertainty within *Renegotiating the Relationship* focused on questioning one's commitment to caregiving, the rules and expectations of the relationship given the PWA's illness, and appropriate strategies for interpersonal conflict with someone who may die soon.

At the outset of illness or the diagnosis of AIDS, caregivers often faced the fundamental question: "Am I willing to do this?" However, many caregivers did not recall consciously choosing to become a caregiver, and instead naturally assumed the role given the nature of their relationship with the PWA. For some caregivers, the increasing strains and demands associated with caregiving provoked uncertainty about staying in or leaving the relationship. Despite his initial commitment to caregiving, one 24-year-old man questioned whether he could continue caring for his lover and cope with the constant changes in their relationship brought about by AIDS:

> *Like any other relationship, you have your ups and*
> *downs, and sometimes there's more downs than ups . . . maybe*
> *it's better for us to . . . you have to decide whether it's healthier*
> *to be in a relationship or healthier to not be in a relationship*
> *. . . I've wanted to end the relationship a number of times, but*
> *then again, I say to myself, take some time, you're overreact-*
> *ing, and say maybe he is doing this because he's dealing with*
> *the whole bit and you have to look at it from that respect.*

Going Public

This category is defined as managing social relationships and choosing social identification based on information about oneself that is both private and very important. Stages and strategies include (a) Living with secrecy, (b) Asserting oneself, and (c) Balancing risks and benefits. The private and important information focused on the caregiver's involvement with the PWA, and, consequently, his or her association with AIDS. The intent of living with secrecy about one's caregiver status was to protect oneself and the PWA from negative judgements, rejection, ridicule, and discriminatory acts. Because these consequences could be devastating, caregivers had a vested interest in anticipating others' responses and in planning accordingly.

The uncertainty of *Going Public* involved the inability to predict others' reactions to the knowledge that the caregiver was taking care of a person with AIDS. One mother felt apprehensive about responding to commonplace inquiries from friends and acquaintances:

> *I really do have a child who is involved in homosexual-*
> *ity, perhaps, and that is not socially acceptable yet. How do I*
> *deal with this? . . . My daughter brought this out just last week,*

and I haven't resolved this issue yet. What am I going to do
when I meet a former neighbor or somebody in a grocery store
who asks, "How are the kids?"

Because of their inability to predict the reactions of others, caregivers often
orchestrated disclosure by carefully choosing who to tell, by making concrete plans
for disclosure, and by staging the type and amount of information given. One
woman spent a considerable amount of time with her friend developing a plan
about how together they would inform his family:

> *His mother had a lot of problems with homosexuality and*
> *with his having AIDS. The day before we started telling his*
> *family we had structured a whole process of how he would in-*
> *form the family, who he would tell first. [We would] sort of*
> *gain acceptance on the most promising ground and move*
> *through a process. And we had this in place, a plan . . .*

Containing the Spread of HIV

This subcategory is defined as the fear surrounding the spread of HIV infection and
the strategies used to prevent transmission to self and others. Stages and strategies
include (a) Confronting fear and personal vulnerability and (b) Doing things differently. Uncertainty about transmission was particularly troubling in the beginning of
caregiving. One priest caring for a close friend in a congregate living setting described the initial questions of the group about *Containing the Spread* in response
to the PWA's move into the house:

> *What do we do with this kind of thing? What does it*
> *mean that he's in the public areas of our house? All the fears*
> *of AIDS. What does a person with AIDS have to watch out for*
> *in terms of hygiene and all those kinds of things? We had a*
> *meeting in which everyone [living in the house] sat down and*
> *talked to each other about it.*

Furthermore, some caregivers lacked confidence in the efficacy of preventive
measures and were not always reassured by scientific information alone. One wife
caring for her husband expressed her mistrust of "safer sex," and had great difficulty resuming their sexual relationship:

> *I know that when I tried to have sex with him I was very*
> *fearful. Even though there was protection and everybody told*
> *me I was 98% safe, I had fear mixed with a lack of trust, and*
> *the whole situation was a great conflict for me.*

One lesbian who was caring for her former lover emphasized the particular
uncertainty associated with female-to-female transmission:

> *I used to always wear gloves during sex and now I don't wear*
> *them sometimes. And the rubber dams, just forget it. I go on*
> *an intuitive basis pretty much. I really make sure I don't have*
> *any cuts on me. I'm a total guinea pig. Nobody knows how*
> *women are going to transfer it.*

For many partners and spouses, an essential component of confronting fear and vulnerability was facing their own HIV status. Many worried about their own HIV exposure, and uncertainty resurfaced each time they sought periodic AIDS testing. One gay partner described the conflict associated with regular HIV testing:

> *It was funny because I got the results of my latest HIV test, and*
> *the next day I flew out of Seattle [on business]. And I'm think-*
> *ing, God, what if this is positive? But it wasn't, thank God . . .*
> *And then, once I got the results of the first test back you feel*
> *like, I'll live forever. But that doesn't mean a year down the*
> *road you won't be. "Oh, no, I thought I was going to escape . . ."*

▧ DISCUSSION

Chick and Meleis (1986) identified illness, recovery, and loss (all of which are integral to the AIDS family caregiving phenomenon) as precipitators of transitions. According to Murphy (1990, p. 1), "A transitions perspective is valuable because, to the extent that transitions are anticipatory, preparation for role change and prevention of negative effects can be instituted." Although most authors equate transitions with change, work by Golan (1981) supports the interrelationship between transitions and uncertainty found in this study; she defined transitions as "a period of moving from one state of certainty to another, with an interval of uncertainty and change in between" (p. 12).

Uncertainty has been studied primarily in relation to experiences with chronic or life-threatening illnesses (Mishel, 1988; Mishel & Braden, 1987; Mishel & Braden, 1988; Cohen, 1989), and more recently pregnancy (Sorenson, 1990), breast cancer (Hilton, 1988), and AIDS (Gordon & Shontz, 1990; Weitz, 1989). In a hermeneutical inquiry that examined living with the AIDS virus, Gordon and Shontz (1990) identified uncertainty as a major theme which was closely woven into the other themes of feeling infected and infectious, facing death and dying, secrecy, and ambivalence. Weitz (1989) found that uncertainty in the lives of PWAs focused on the acquisition of AIDS, the meaning of symptoms, short-term functioning, living with dignity, and the prognosis of AIDS. Given the uncertainty experienced by PWAs, it is not surprising that similar concerns regarding uncertainty were prevalent among family members in this study.

While uncertainty has been noted in other caregiving situations, such as cancer, it is a relatively unexplored theme in the family caregiving literature. Research about caregiver uncertainty suggests (a) an association between uncertainty and caregiver health (Stetz, 1989), (b) uncertainty related to the course of therapy and outcomes resulted in significant caregiver needs (Blank, Clark, Longman, & Atwood, 1989), (c) uncertainty associated with managing the illness and monitoring symptoms was a significant source of stress for parents of chronically ill children (Cohen, 1989), and (d) the early stages of caregiving for the cognitively impaired elderly were marked with uncertainty and unpredictability (Wilson, 1989). Much of the uncertainty in the family caregiving literature was associated with the illness itself, whereas data in the present study revealed that uncertainty in AIDS caregiving also pertained to loss and dying, interpersonal relationships, contagion, and the presentation of self. Furthermore, uncertainty was an important concern for caregivers, similar to the uncertainty reported by family members of cancer patients (Chekryn, 1985; Germino, 1984).

The results advance understanding of AIDS caregiving uncertainty by integrating a theoretical perspective on transitions, by delineating cultural and social contextual features, and by specifying content areas (that is, according to the five caregiving subcategories). Therefore, the findings highlight directions for developing clinical therapeutics in the areas of AIDS family caregiving and uncertainty. Anticipatory guidance could be an important strategy to help caregivers cope with uncertainty because they can identify it, expect it, accept it, and define which of the uncertain circumstances are appropriate and desirable to change. Anticipating caregiving as a transitional period marked by major changes and a new perspective on what is important in life may help reduce the strain associated with the demands of caregiving. In considering clinical therapeutics for AIDS family caregivers, significant gaps remain in understanding the content and timing of the most appropriate interventions. Longitudinal research designs are best suited to address these gaps because of the transitional nature of caregiving as it changes over time. Longitudinal data about AIDS family caregiving are essential to refine the content and timing of interventions, to maximize therapeutic value, and to enhance cost-effectiveness.

▨ REFERENCES

Baumgarten, M. (1989). The health of a person giving care to the demented elderly: A critical review of literature. *Journal of Clinical Epidemiology, 42,* 1137–1148.

Blank, J. J., Clark, L., Longman, A. J., & Atwood, J. R. (1989). Perceived home care needs of cancer patients and their caregivers. *Cancer Nursing, 12*(2), 78–84.

Blumer, H. (1969). *Symbolic interactionism: Perspective and method.* Englewood Cliffs, NJ: Prentice Hall.

Bowers, B. (1987). Intergenerational caregiving: Adult caregivers and their aging parents. *Advances in Nursing Science, 9*(2), 20–31.

Chekryn, J. (1984). Cancer recurrence: Personal meaning, communication and marital adjustment. *Cancer Nursing, 7,* 491–498.

Chenoweth, B., & Spencer, B. (1986). Dementia: The experience of family caregivers. *The Gerontologist, 26,* 267–272.

Chick, N., & Meleis, A. I. (1986). Transitions: A nursing concern. In P. L. Chinn (Ed.), *Nursing research methodology* (pp. 237–257). Rockville, MD: Aspen.

Cohen, M. H. (1989). The sources and management of uncertainty in life-threatening chronic illness [Abstract]. *Communicating Nursing Research, 22,* 155.

DSHS & Seattle-King County Health Department. (1991). *Washington St/Seattle-King County HIV/AIDS Epidemiology Report,* 1st quarter, p. 1.

Edwards, B. (1988). Stories from the front: How to cope when your lover has ARC or AIDS. In T. Eidson (Ed.), *The AIDS caregiver's handbook* (pp. 206–216). New York: St. Martin's Press.

Ekberg, J., Griffith, N., & Foxall, M. J. (1986). Spouse burnout syndrome. *Journal of Advanced Nursing, 1,* 161–165.

Germino, B. B. (1984). *Family members' concerns after cancer diagnosis.* Unpublished doctoral dissertation, University of Washington, Seattle.

Glaser, B., & Strauss, A. (1967). *The discovery of grounded theory: Strategies for qualitative research.* Chicago: Aldine.

Golan, N. (1981). *Passing through transitions.* New York: Free Press.

Gordon, J., & Shontz, F. (1990). Living with the AIDS virus: A representative case. *Journal of Counseling and Development, 68,* 287–292.

Haque, R. (1989). A family's experience with AIDS. In J. H. Flaskerud (Ed.), *AIDS/HIV Infection: A reference guide for nursing professionals* (pp. 230–240). Philadelphia: W. B. Saunders.

Hepburn, K. (1990). Informal caregivers: Front-line workers in the chronic care of AIDS patients. In *Community based care for persons with AIDS: Developing a research agenda* (pp. 37–42), (DHHS Publication No. (PHS) 90-3456). Washington, DC: U.S. Government Printing Office.

Hilton, B. A. (1988). The phenomenon of uncertainty in women with breast cancer. *Issues in Mental Health Nursing, 9,* 217–238.

Lincoln, Y. S., & Guba, E. G. (1985). *Naturalistic inquiry.* Beverly Hills, CA: Sage.

Livingston, M. (1985). Families who care. *British Medical Journal, 291,* 919–920.

Miller, B., & Montgomery, A. (1990). Family caregivers and limitations in social activities. *Research on Aging, 12,* 72–93.

Mishel, M. (1990). Reconceptualization of the Uncertainty in Illness Theory. *IMAGE: Journal of Nursing Scholarship, 22,* 256–262.

Mishel, M. (1988). Uncertainty in illness. *Image, 20,* 225–232.

Mishel, M., & Braden, C. (1987). Uncertainty: A mediator between support and adjustment. *Western Journal of Nursing Research, 9,* 43–57.

Mishel, M., & Braden, M. (1988). Finding meaning: Antecedents of uncertainty in illness. *Nursing Research, 37,* 98–103.

Moffatt, B. C. (1986). *When someone you love has AIDS.* New York: NAL Penguin.

Monette, P. (1988). *Borrowed time.* New York: Avon Books.

Montgomery, R., Gonyea, J., & Hooyman, N. (1985). Caregiving and the experience of subjective and objective burden. *Family Relations, 34,* 19–26.

Murphy, S. A. (1990). Human responses to transitions: A holistic nursing perspective. *Holistic Nursing Practice, 4*(3), 1–7.

Ostrow, D., & Gayle, T. (1986). Psychosocial and ethical issues of AIDS health care programs. *Quarterly Review Bulletin, 12,* 284–294.

Parkes, C. M. (1971). Psycho-social transitions: A field for study. *Social Science & Medicine, 5,* 101–115.

Rabins, P. V., Mace, N. L., & Lucas, M. J. (1982). The impact of dementia on the family. *Journal of the American Medical Association, 248,* 333–335.

Rabins, P. V., Fitting, M. D., Eastham, J., & Fetting, J. (1990). The emotional impact of caring for the chronically ill. *Psychosomatics, 31,* 331–336.

Raveis, V., & Siegel, K. (1990). Impact of caregiving on informal or familial caregivers. In *Community-based care of persons with AIDS: Developing a research agenda* (pp. 17–28). (DHHS Publication Number (PHS) 90-3456). Washington, DC: U.S. Printing Office.

Sandelowski, M. (1986). The problem of rigor in qualitative research. *Advances in Nursing Science, 8*(3), 27–37.

Schoen, K. (1986). Psychosocial aspects of hospice care for AIDS patients. *The American Journal of Hospice Care, 3*(2), 32–34.

Shilts, R. (1987). *And the band played on: Politics, people, and the AIDS epidemic.* New York: St. Martin's Press.

Snyder, B., & Keefe, K. (1985). The unmet needs of family caregivers for frail and disabled adults. *Social Work in Health Care, 10*(3), 1–14.

Sorenson, D. (1990). Uncertainty in pregnancy. NAACOG's *Clinical Issues in Perinatal and Women's Health Nursing, 1,* 289–296.

Stetz, K. (1989). The relationship among background characteristics, purpose in life, and caregiving demands on perceived health of spouse caregivers. *Scholarly Inquiry for Nursing Practice, 3,* 133–159.

Strauss, A. L. (1987). *Qualitative analysis for social scientists.* Cambridge: Cambridge University Press.

Thomas, R. (1987). Family adaptation to a child with a chronic condition. In M. H. Rose & R. B. Thomas (Eds.). *Children with chronic conditions* (pp. 29–54). New York: Harcourt Brace Jovanovich.

Weitz, R. (1989). Uncertainty and the lives of persons with AIDS. *Journal of Health and Social Behavior, 30,* 270–281.

Wilson, H. S. (1989). Family caregiving for a relative with Alzheimer's dementia: Coping with negative choices. *Nursing Research, 38,* 94–98.

Wolcott, D. L. Fawzy, F. I., Landsverk, J., & McCombs, M. (1986). AIDS patients' needs of psychosocial services and their use of community service organizations. *Journal of Psychosocial Oncology, 4,* 135–146.

Zarit, S. H., Todd, P. A., & Zarit, J. M. (1986). Subjective burden of husbands and wives as caregivers. A longitudinal study. *The Gerontologist, 26,* 260–266.

Appendix
Answers to Selected Study Guide Exercises

Chapter 1

A.1.   1a 2c 3c 4c 5a 6b 7c 8b 9c 10d

A.2.   1a 2b 3d 4a 5b 6a 7b 8d 9b 10c 11a 12a

B.   1. Florence Nightingale   2. Nursing education   3. 1950s   4. Clinical practice
5. Tradition   6. Inductive   7. Determinism   8. Naturalistic   9. Scientific   10. Empirical   11. Generalization   12. Reductionist   13. Field   14. Quantitative research   15. Qualitative research   16. Identification

C.7.   a. Basic   b. Applied   c. Applied   d. Basic   e. Basic   f. Applied   g. Basic
h. Applied

Chapter 2

A.1.   1a 2c 3b 4a 5b 6a 7c 8c

A.2.   1a 2b 3c 4b 5a 6a 7b 8c 9a 10b 11a 12b

A.3.   1b 2c 3b 4a 5b 6c 7c 8c

B.   1. Principal investigator, project director   2. Subjects, study participants
3. Concepts   4. Variable   5. Categorical   6. Independent   7. Dependent
8. Independent   9. Data   10. Operational definitions   11. Qualitative   12. Patterns of association   13. Causal (cause-and-effect)   14. Functional   15. Qualitative, quantitative   16. Quantitative   17. Research design   18. Sample   19. Empirical (data collection)   20. Data analysis   21. Pilot study   22. Research reports, journal articles   23. Dissemination   24. Gaining entrée   25. Saturation
26. Abstract, introduction, method, results, discussion, references

C.   3 and C.4[1]

Independent	*Dependent*
a. Participation/nonparticipation in assertiveness training (categorical)	Nursing effectiveness (continuous)
b. Patients' postural positioning (categorical)	Respiratory function (continuous)
c. Amount of touch by nursing staff (continuous)	Patients' psychological well-being (continuous)
d. Frequency of turning patients (continuous)	Incidence of decubitus (continuous)
e. Educational preparation of nurses (categorical)	Turnover rate (continuous)
f. Patients' age (continuous) and gender (categorical)	Tolerance for pain (continuous)
g. Number of prenatal visits (continuous)	Labor and delivery outcomes (continuous—*e.g.,* length of time in labor; or categorical—*e.g.,* vaginal versus cesarean delivery)
h. Pediatric versus adult intensive care unit (ICU) assignment (categorical)	Nurses' stress levels (continuous)
i. Student nurses' clinical grades (continuous)	On-the-job performance (continuous)
j. Method of preoperative teaching (categorical)	Anxiety levels of patients (continuous)
k. Level of participation in continuing education activities (continuous)	Nurses' promotions (categorical)
l. Time of day (continuous)	Hearing acuity among the elderly (continuous)
m. Congruity of nurses' and patients' cultural backgrounds (categorical)	Patient satisfaction with nursing care (continuous)
n. Women's educational backgrounds (continuous)	Breast self-examination practices (categorical)
o. Setting of childbirth: home versus hospital (categorical)	Parents' satisfaction with childbirth experience (continuous)

---

[1]For some of these variables, there is no absolutely correct answer with regard to whether the variable is categorical or continuous since it would depend on the operational definition established by the researcher. For example, in Question C.3(n), the educational background of women could be measured as a continuous variable (number of years of schooling completed) or as a categorical variable (did not complete high school versus completed high school). Since researchers can always collapse continuous variables into categorical variables, we have indicated those variables that *could* be continuous as continuous variables.

Chapter 3

A.1. 1b 2c 3a 4b 5a 6c 7b 8a

A.2. 1a 2c 3d 4a 5b 6d 7a 8c 9b 10d 11b 12c 13b 14a 15c

B. 1. Research problem 2. Research question 3 Research aims, objectives 4. Experience, literature, social issues, theory, external sources 5. Qualitative 6. Unfeasible 7. Unresearchable 8. Introduction 9. Relationship 10. Two 11. Multivariate (complex) 12. Null (statistical)

Independent	*Dependent*
4a. Clinical specialty area	Attitudes toward mental retardation
4b. Nurses versus patients	Perceived importance of attending to physical versus emotional needs
4c. Type of nursing care (Primary versus team nursing)	Patient satisfaction with nursing care
4d. Frequency of turning	Incidence of decubitus ulcers
4e. Type of nursing preparation (baccalaureate versus associate program)	Use of therapeutic touch
5a. Number of prior blood donations	Stress
5b. Nurses' frequency of initiating conversation	Patients' ratings of nursing effectiveness
5c. Patients' ratings of nurses' informativeness	Degree of preoperative stress
5d. Draining versus no draining of peritoneum	Incidence of infection
5e. Method of delivery (cesarean versus vaginal)	Incidence of postpartum depression

Chapter 4

A.1. 1c 2e 3d 4e 5d 6a 7b 8d

A.2. 1c 2d 3f 4a 5e 6b

B. 1. CINAHL 2. Subject 3. Textword 4. Indexes, abstract journals 5. Primary 6. Opinions, anecdotes 7. Findings from other research 8. Relevance 9. Quotes 10. Gaps 11. Critical summary 12. Tentativeness 13. Introduction, discussion 14. Framework 15. Invented (created, constructed) 16. Conceptual models (frameworks, schemes) 17. Words 18. Person, environment, health, nursing 19. Health Promotion Model 20. Borrowed theories

Chapter 5

A.1.   1d 2b 3c 4b 5a 6d 7b 8a 9c 10a 11b 12d

B.1.   Dilemmas   2. Nuremberg code   3. *Belmont Report*   4. Harm   5. Minimal risks   6. Self-determination   7. Full disclosure   8. Anonymity   9. Vulnerable 10. Institutional Review Boards

Chapter 6

A.1.   1b 2b 3a 4d 5b 6a 7d 8a 9b, c 10d

A.2.   1a, d 2c 3a 4b 5d 6b 7a 8b

B.   1. Experimental, nonexperimental   2. Comparison   3. Independent 4. Treatment (intervention)   5. Systematic bias   6. Pretest   7. Factorial design 8. Levels   9. Double blind   10. Repeated measures   11. Causality (cause-and-effect relationships)   12. Comparison   13. Preexperimental   14. Time series 15. Equivalent   (equal)   16. Nonexperimental   17. Independent 18. Causal (cause and effect)   19. Retrospective   20. Longitudinal   21. Follow-up studies   22. Surveys   23. Evaluation   24. Key informant   25. Methods 26. Constancy   27. Generalizability   28. Internal   29. Mortality   30. Maturation

C.2.   a. Cannot   b. Can   c. Can   d. Cannot   e. Cannot   f. Cannot   g. Can h. Cannot   i. Can   j. Can   k. Cannot   l. Can   m. Can   n. Cannot   o. Can

C.5.   4.a. Nonexperimental   4.b. Nonexperimental   4.c. Both   4.d. Both 4.e. Nonexperimental   5.a. Nonexperimental   5.b. Both   5.c. Nonexperimental 5.d. Both   5.e. Nonexperimental

Chapter 7

A.1.   1b 2a 3d 4a 5b 6a 7b 8c 9d 10c

A.2.   2c 2a 3c 4d 5c 6a 7c 8a

B.   1. Anthropology, psychology, sociology   2. Cultures   3. Researcher as instrument   4. Essence   5. Spatiality,   corporeality,   temporality,   relationality 6. Grounded theory   7. Complementary   8. Validity

C.2.   a. Grounded theory   b. Ethnography   c. Discourse analysis   d. Phenomenology

Chapter 8

A.1.   1b   2c   3a   4b   5b   6c   7a   8a   9d   10b

A.2.   1c   2a   3d   4b   5c   6b   7c   8d   9a   10d

B.   1. Sample   2. Representativeness   3. Biased   4. Homogeneous   5. Accidental sample   6. Strata   7. Judgmental; purposeful; theoretical   8. Simple random sampling   9. Weighting   10. Multistage   11. Sampling interval   12. Sampling error   13. Accessible   14. Increases   15. 30   16. Information   17. Homogeneous; maximum variation   18. Typical case

C.2.   a. Multistage (cluster)   b. Convenience (accidental)   c. Simple random   d. Systematic   e. Quota   f. Extreme (deviant) case   g. Snowball (network)

C.3.   Sampling interval = 22; elements = 134, 156, 178

Chapter 9

A.1.   1b   2a   3c   4c   5d   6a   7b   8c

A.2.   1c   2b   3a   4a   5a   6b   7b   8a   9c   10a

B.   1. Existing data   2. Historical research   3. Secondary analysis   4. Structure, quantifiability, researcher obtrusiveness, objectivity   5. Topic guide   6. Focus group interview   7. Closed-ended (fixed-alternative)   8. Open-ended   9. Pretest   10. Closed-ended (fixed alternative)   11. Scale   12. Declarative   13. Reversed   14. Bipolar adjectives   15. Extreme response set   16. Response set biases   17. Vignettes   18. Behavior   19. Reactivity   20. Participant observation   21. Single, multiple, mobile   22. Logs, field notes   23. Category system   24. In vivo   25. In vitro

C.3.   Y = 11; Z = 26

C.4.   A = Acquiescence   B = None   C = Extreme response set   D = Nay-sayers' bias

C.5.   a5   b1   c1   d5   e5   f1   g5   h5   i5   j1
Minimum score = 10, maximum score = 50

Chapter 10

A.1.   1a 2c 3b 4c 5a 6d 7b 8a

A.2.   1a 2c 3b 4d 5a 6b

B.   1. Attributes (characteristics)   2. Quantification   3. Rules   4. True score
5. Measurement error   6. True score   7. Stability   8. Split-half   9. Homogeneity
10. Interrater (interobserver) reliability   11. Valid   12. Face   13. Content
14. Predictive   15. Credibility, transferability, dependability, confirmability
16. Prolonged engagement   17. Data triangulation   18. Member checking
19. Confirmability   20. Inquiry audit

Chapter 11

A.1.   1d 2a 3d 4b 5c 6a 7b 8d 9c 10b 11c 12a

A.2.   1b 2a 3c 4c 5d 6b 7b 8a 9c 10a

A.3.   1b 2a 3d 4b 5c 6a 7a 8a 9d 10c

A.4.   1a, b, d 2a 3c 4e 5a, b, c, d, e 6b, d 7d 8e

B.   1. Enumeration (count)   2. Ordinal   3. Zero   4. Equal distances   5. Param-
eter   6. Frequency distribution   7. Frequency polygons   8. Symmetric   9. Negatively   10. Unimodal   11. Normal curve (bell-shaped curve)   12. Central tendency   13. Variability   14. Homogeneous   15. Standard deviation   16. Bivariate
statistics   17. Negative (inverse)   18. Pearson's r (product—moment correlation
coefficient)   19. Inferential statistics   20. Normal   21. Type I   22. Parametric
23. Levels of significance   24. Type II   25. F-ratio   26. Chi-squared test   27. R
28. Analysis of covariance   29. Covariate   30. Factors   31. Factor extraction
phase   32. Multivariate analysis of variance

C.3.   Unimodal, fairly symmetric

C.4.   Mean: 81.13;   Median: 83;   Mode: 84

C.7.   a. Chi-squared   b. t-test   c. Pearson's r d. ANOVA

C.9.   a. Discriminant function analysis or logistic regression   b. ANCOVA
c. MANOVA   d. Multiple regression

Chapter 12

A.   1a 2d 3c 4a 5b 6b

B.   1. Simultaneously   2. Comprehending, synthesizing, theorizing, recontextualizing   3. Indexing, categorizing   4. Constant comparison   5. Open coding (Level I coding)   6. Conceptual file   7. Computer programs   8. Themes   9. Quasi-statistics   10. Analytic induction   11. Axial coding   12. Basic social process

Chapter 13

A.1.   1b 2c 3b 4d 5b 6a 7d 8c 9a 10a

A.2.   1b 2c 3d 4b 5b 6a 7c 8d

B.   1. Accuracy   2. Hypothesis   3. Causation   4. Their data   5. Important (useful)   6. Decisions   7. Strengths, weaknesses (virtues, flaws)   8. Substantive/theoretical   9. Methodologic   10. Ethical   11. Interpretive   12. Stylistic/presentational

Chapter 14

A.1.   1b (also c)   2a 3c 4a 5a (also b and c)   6b (also a and c)   7c 8c 9b (also c)   10b (also a and c)

B.   1. Research utilization   2. Gap   3. Conduct and Utilization Research in Nursing (CURN)   4. Western Interstate Commission for Higher Education (WICHE) Regional Program for Nursing Research Development   5. Replicated   6. Implementation potential   7. Transferability   8. The cost/benefit of *not* implementing it